1

NEGATIVE THOUGHTS DON'T HAVE TO OWN YOU:
Enhance Your Career and Improve Your Health

By
Vivian Orgel

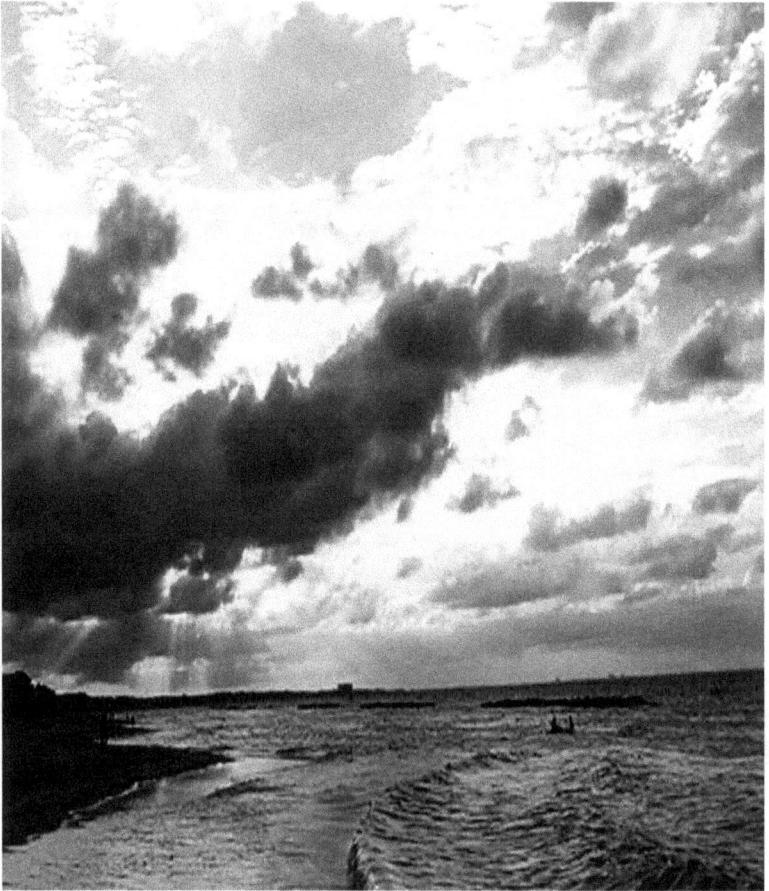

"You Either Grow Wise or Otherwise."
— Vivian Orgel

Copyright

Library of Congress cataloging in publication data
www.VivianOrgel.com
ISBN ebook 978-1-931403-26-9
ISBN All full Color 978-1-931403-34-4
ISBN Color and Black and white version
Published by M.B.B.C., INC. 2019

Disclaimer

The entire content herein is based on the opinions of Vivian Orgel and MBBC, Inc., unless otherwise noted. Individual articles are based on research and the opinions and experiences of the author, who retains copyright privileges as marked. The information herein and on Vivian Orgel's website is not intended to replace a one-on-one relationship with a qualified healthcare professional and is not intended as medical advice. It is intended as a sharing of knowledge, information, research and experience by Ms.

Orgel, with her community. Ms. Orgel encourages you to make your own healthcare decisions based on your research and in partnership with a qualified healthcare professional.

Learn Why It's Not Your Fault

Also, How to:

- Overcome Negativity, Like I Have Every Day.

- Embrace What Can Change Your Life.

- Take Simple Action Steps to Free Yourself.

- Enhance Your Life and Your Career, Through Overcoming Negativity.

- Understand the Mind-Body Connection.

- Recognize the Symptoms and Causes of Negativity.

- Challenge Obstacles, So You Can Benefit from Them.

- Discover the Person You Want to Be.

- Let Blessings Unfold.

- Improve Your Overall Health and Appearance.

- Get Through It All.

About the Author

Vivian Orgel is a pioneer of advancements in beauty, health and well-being. She focuses on strategies for stress reeducation and safety. Her extensive research sheds light on expert advice from many world-renowned healthcare professionals who are dedicated to emotional well-being and skin injury prevention, care and renewal.

Vivian Orgel brings medical attention to underlying causes of skin injuries, poor healing, unwanted hair growth and prevention in interviews found in articles published by *Dermascope: The Encyclopedia of Aesthetics and Spa Therapy* and consumer magazines, including *GQ, Glamour, Vogue, Self, Seventeen* and *Essence*—also in articles and books she has published herself.

VISIT Vivian's website at **www.VivianOrgel.com** for more on how she integrates self-care, self-protection and vital strategies for better health and well-being.

TABLE OF CONTENTS

PART I

INTRODUCTION

"You Either Grow Wise or Otherwise.
If inventors like Edison had stopped,
we would all be in the dark
—Vivian Orgel

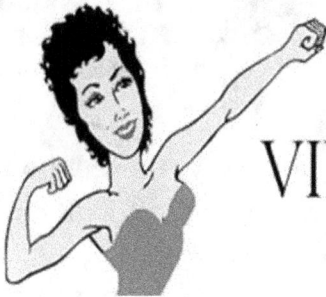

VIVIAN • ORGEL
FOR LIFE'S CHALLENGES

CHAPTER 1

INVITATION TO GROW WISER

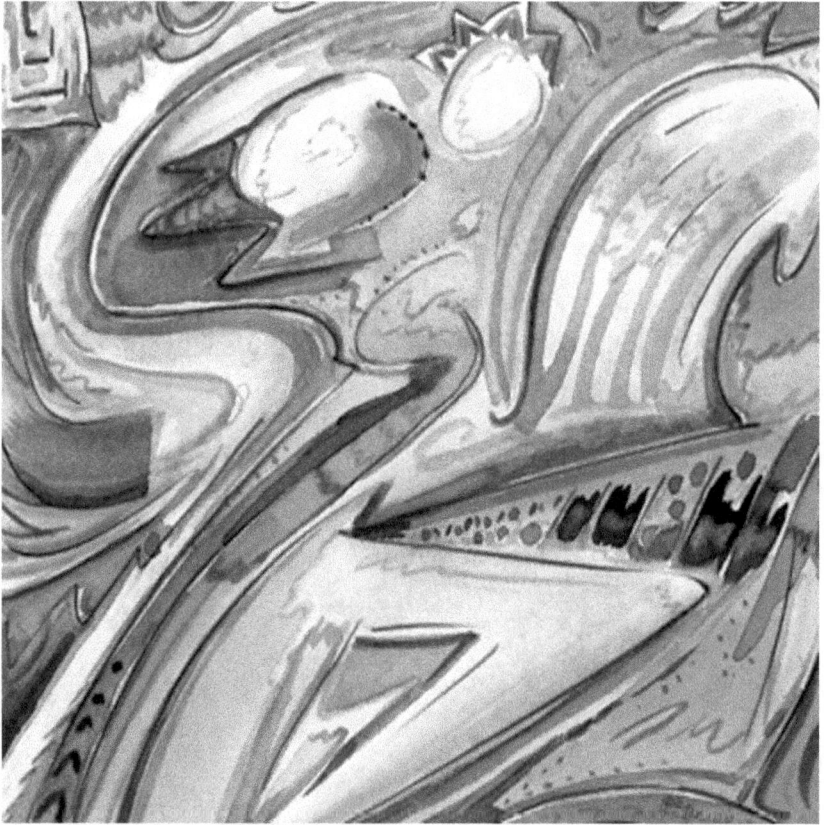

Henry Brown

"In spite of discouragement and adversity, those who are happiest seem to have a way of learning from difficult times, becoming stronger, wiser and happier as a result."

— Joseph B. Wirthlin

This book is my invitation to you to join me in my journey toward becoming more **positive** and, therefore, happier, wiser and more **productive** every day. In it, I share with you what has helped me move through and beyond traumatic experiences that could have negatively impacted my life, had I not recognized their power and potential to harm me and not chosen to confront them and do what was needed to counteract their influence.

I share three milestones in my life as examples of how I used positive thinking and actions to overcome their negative power. The first has to do with my childhood upbringing; the second was how, as an adult, I was deceived by a financial Ponzi scheme and, more recently, how a fire destroyed my home.

Not long ago, I invested a lot of money in a company that scammed me and 1,399 other people. Because of the actions I took, other investors **benefited**, and I also **gained** an overall sense of confidence and well-being, having not been left feeling powerless. Those actions also put me in a better position to help even more people with my fraud prevention book: *An Eye-opening Insider Investment Scam Report for Consumers,* something I never would have written, had I allowed myself to get stuck in negativity and defeat. By choosing a positive reaction to my misfortune, I was able to turn a bad situation into a **money-making** venture, including presenting keynote lectures on this topic.

Soon after being victimized by the Ponzi scheme, I was hit with yet another unexpected disaster—an electrical fire gutted my apartment!

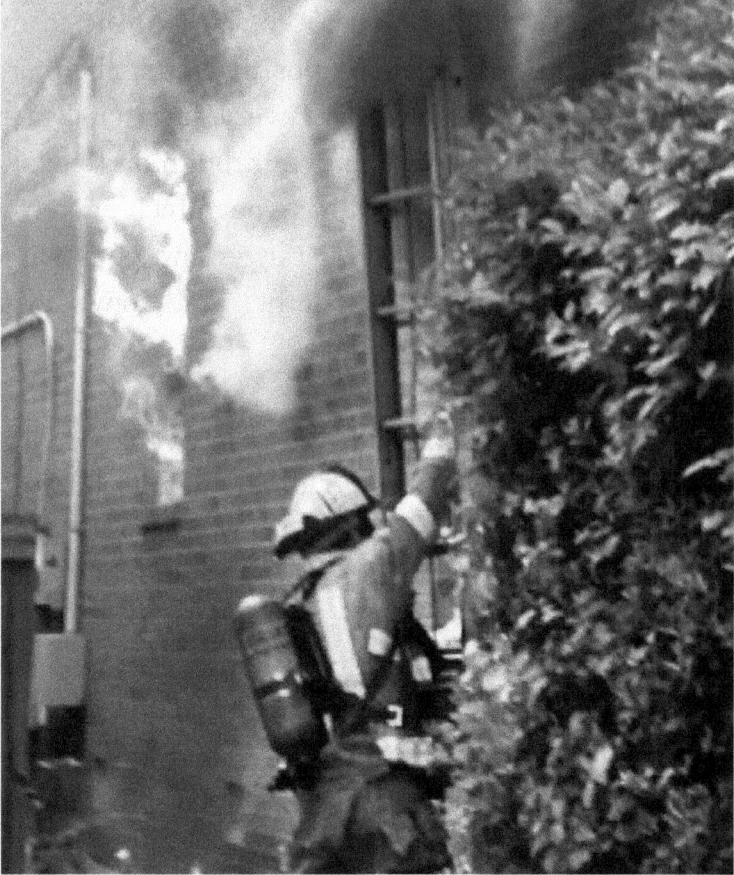

From this catastrophe, I learned several valuable life lessons. During the following ten months, I lived out of shopping bags and in four different apartments. The building restoration taught me a lot about how to keep myself calm, while going through stressful, uncomfortable circumstances.

I never talk about this next topic, but a couple of weeks ago, I listened to an Oprah Winfrey interview on *60 Minutes* about childhood trauma and realized I didn't know any of my friends or clients that had been through this.

I had talked about my childhood being a negative experience, but, maybe for my own self-protection, I had never thought of it as being traumatic.

Looking back, I remember I was always making things and going after things. All the frequent beatings I had endured were tucked so far away that I didn't think of that abuse at all, until my 68-year-old cousin sparked my memory. She reminded me that she had been in the basement and had seen and heard my dad beating me.

I figured out a long time ago that my upbringing caused me to experience low self-esteem. An overall lack of communication was the norm in my household, where there was never a meaningful connection with my parents. Because I didn't experience what it was like to be loved or cared for when I was growing up, I always felt less worthy than others and looked to the world around me to tell me I was okay.

That was then. Now I am self-empowered. I worked my way into a career that allowed me to help others. While working as an electrologist and director of hair removal at Bloomingdale's, I was fortunate enough to be surrounded and influenced by strong women. Through that experience and learning how to heal myself, I became an advocate for consumers who sought more natural solutions to health, beauty and well-being. My need and determination to advocate for myself and others started my journey.

After seeing the interview with Oprah, I felt it could help give us all a better understanding of others' behaviors, feelings and beliefs and how low self-esteem and more serious problems can result from living through a traumatic childhood. I overcame my negative childhood, because I wanted a better life. YOU CAN DO THIS AS WELL.

These negative milestones in my life had the potential to put me into a long-lasting negative frame of mind. However, I chose the path to positivity and to see all the events in my life as learning experiences. I could have chosen to perceive them as negative events, with power to affect my life in a terrible way. I chose, instead, to tap into what is available to us all—the ability to change our perspective.

I've been knocked down for the count several times in my life, nevertheless, like Rocky, I get back up. My ability to overcome and find a positive side to these disasters is evidence that, even in the midst of a catastrophe, you can always learn something that can help you in the future.

You should never underestimate the power of positive thinking. It not only benefits your emotional, but also your physical, **well-being**. Positive thinking is about learning and choosing to focus on your **strengths,** while still being aware of your weaknesses. **Optimistic** people believe good things are long-lasting and the norm; they benefit from almost everything that happens in their lives, and they view bad events as isolated and temporary. As a result, positive thinkers feel **powerful**, whereas negative thinkers feel helpless. *This feeling of helplessness is a major factor contributing to depression and stress.*

As a plus, positive thinkers live longer. Studies show that even the elderly suffering from ailments, can extend their lives and quality of life through **optimism**. Those who don't let the crippling ailments defeat them, continue to get the most out of life that they can. This is because positive emotions regulate and decrease the effects negative emotions have on our well-being.

Although negativity can stunt your growth, I'm here to help you understand that, no matter how devastating and overwhelming the circumstances, you can overcome them through positivity.

I am sharing my knowledge and experience with you, to give you hope that you can overcome a negative past or current circumstance, as I have. Feeling generally happier and more **confident** about our lives, is what this book is all about.

Nothing I'm sharing with you is in any way meant to make you feel bad about negative thinking. It's not your fault, when you are born into a negative environment, and we all get stuck in negative thinking at times—and sometimes for very good reasons. To get out of that rut, we may need someone or something to wake us up and motivate us to do what is needed to get unstuck. **Hopefully**, you are reading this now, because you are ready for that something to get you started.

Please take from this book, including the exercises and suggestions for healing, what you need or find helpful. All are meant to show you how changing your thinking can change your whole life. The information I provide is comprehensive and backed by recent scientific studies. It includes facts about how certain physical conditions, not just problems and past traumas, can get you stuck in negativity. You will be introduced to new technology that can make your brain work better and change the way you perceive reality, which is the key to overcoming negativity. You may come to understand that changing your mind-frame or mood is a lot easier than you thought.

My **hope** is that after you commit to following some or all of the book's suggestions, you will feel **better**, look better, have better control of life's unavoidable challenges and experiences, and achieve, overall, a happier and more **fulfilling** life.

I will first define what negativity is, its causes and effects, and then give suggestions on what can be done to overcome it. At any point that you decide you want to move past the cause and effects and fast-forward to the **Solutions**, just go to that section, and get started. You will notice throughout the book that some **positive words** are printed in bold type, and the reason for this will become clear to you as you read on.

Hopefully as you get a better understanding of how and why negativity dominates your life, you will find solutions here to help you work positively through a lot of your problems, just as I did.

CHAPTER 2

WHAT IS NEGATIVITY?

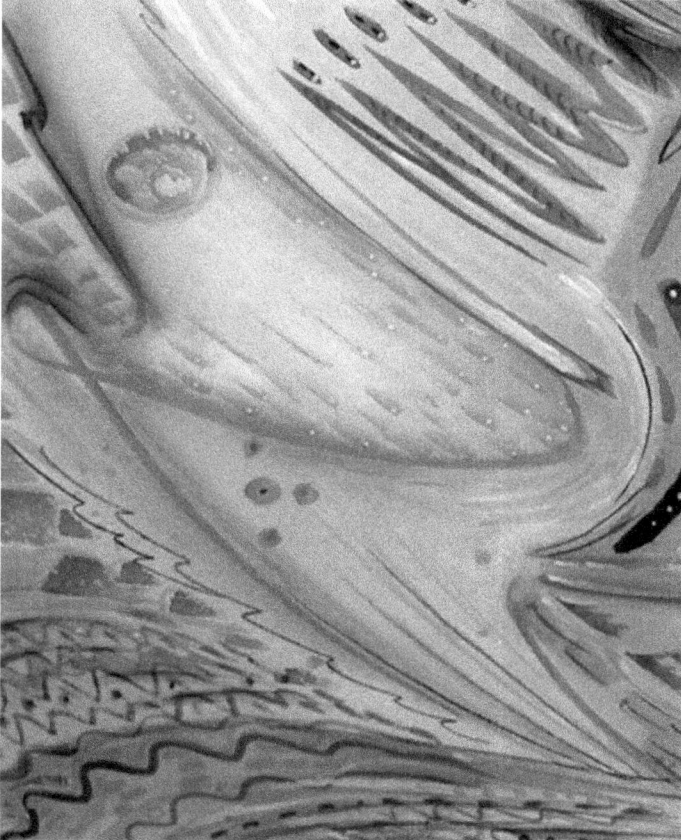

Henry Brown

"Believing in negative thoughts is the single
greatest obstruction to success.
—Charles F. Glassman

To better understand the subject of this book, we first need to talk about what it means to be negative. The Merriam-Webster dictionary defines negative as: "Harmful or bad, not wanted" and also "Experiencing dislike or disapproval."

A well-known expression of negativity is a habit of seeing a half-full glass as half-empty. Negative Thinking, therefore, can be defined as: "Thinking about the bad qualities of someone or something, thinking that a bad result will happen and/or not hopeful or optimistic."

Negativity is not about just having negative thoughts or feelings; it's about rarely having a positive perspective on things that happen—about rarely seeing the **bright** side or the cloud's **"silver lining."**

Studies have found that regularly experiencing a **variety** of emotions, including negative ones, is important to our health. We all need to feel what we really feel and not suppress those emotions. What we want to avoid, however, is getting into a rut, for whatever reason, and developing a tendency to focus on the negative aspect of things and ourselves, others or life, in general, most or all of the time. It can be a very sad and unproductive existence for those stuck in negativity and for those involved in relationships with people who have only or mostly negative perceptions.

Negativity becomes a habit—one that can be very addictive—a habit of thinking negatively, most or all of the time—a habit that can stunt your growth, by obstructing your ability to see the **possibilities** within a challenging situation. When you are focusing on what's wrong, you're blocking **advancement**, opportunities, joy—even blocking **love**.

On the other hand, **positivity** can be defined as: "the practice of being or tendency to be positive or **optimistic** in attitude," which is something that doesn't come naturally or easily for all of us or for humans, in general, for reasons we'll explain later.

If your thoughts are dominated by negativity, it can affect everything you do and say and even the way you look and feel.

BUT THE GOOD NEWS IS: none of this means you can't break out of a negativity rut and live a happier and more fulfilled life.

SIGNS THAT WE'RE STUCK IN NEGATIVITY

Below are some examples of Negative Thoughts, Emotions, Feelings and Actions. See if you can identify with any of the thoughts and feelings, and/or try to recognize if you might have been unconsciously doing any of the actions —or even procrastinating because of negativity. Remember, the concern is not about having these feelings now and then, but about rarely experiencing emotions other than negative thoughts and feelings.

A. Negative Thoughts

- Focusing only on the problem

- Everything bad happens to me.

- I can't help it.

- Over-generalizing (always, never)

- Polarizing (only good or bad)

- Never satisfied

B. Negative Emotions/Feelings

- Jealousy

- Anger/Irritability

- Low self-esteem

- Worthlessness

- Helplessness

- Feeling stuck—in a rut

C. Negative Actions

- Blaming others

- Abusing oneself or others

- Criticizing others, to divert attention from oneself

- Getting and staying stuck in negative patterns or old thinking habits

- Selfishness/Self absorption—it's always about you

- Controlling/Manipulative

D. Negative Inaction

- Procrastination or Paralysis—negative thoughts cause us to put off or keep us from doing what needs to be done or achieving our goals.

CHAPTER 3

CAUSES OF NEGATIVITY

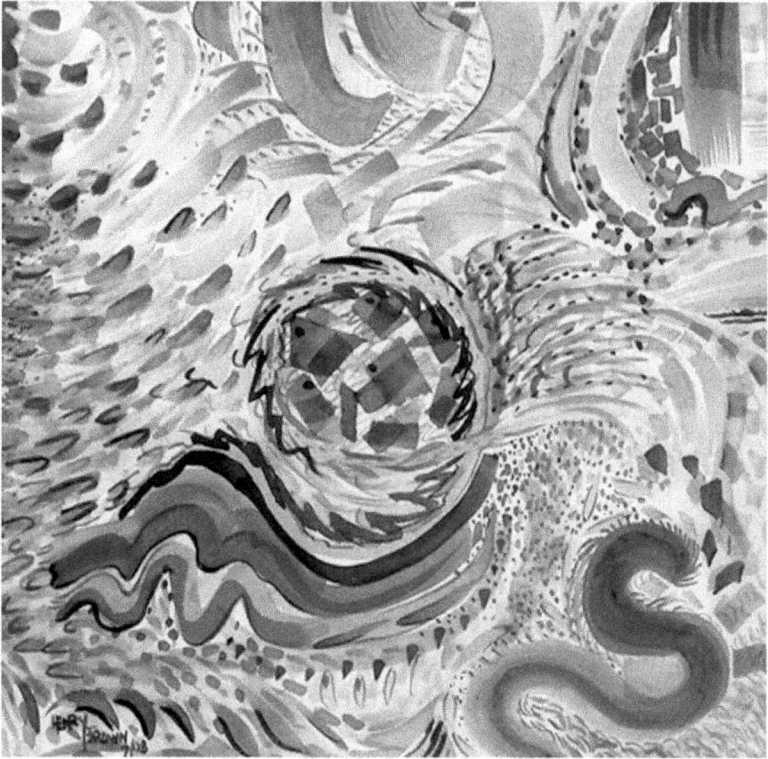

Henry Brown

"It is the mind that maketh good or ill, that maketh
wretch or happy, rich or poor."

— Edmund Spenser

WHY ARE WE NEGATIVE?

It's a great question. But it may take time to find the answer. The reason could be simple. Your negativity might result from your inability to cope with situations, because you're unprepared, or you don't have the information you need. You might easily overcome this, through trying a few tips on preparation and discipline.

Fear might be the source. You could be using negativity as a barrier to keep people away to shield yourself from being hurt. Fear of being hurt can turn into a fear of relationships. Negativity can also be used as an excuse for inaction, and what's behind this is often fear of failure. These types of fear and other fears can be difficult to overcome, but you do not have to allow fear to control you. Instead of allowing it to be a roadblock to progress or happiness, you can choose to view it as merely an obstacle you can move around. You can learn from it and learn to confront it.

Often the cause of negative thinking is much more complex. How we were brought up, can have a profound influence on how we think and act as adults. If you are finding yourself stuck in a negative mindset, you're not alone. It is not uncommon at all for people who have had a difficult childhood or who have suffered some type abuse, to become controlled by negative thinking and stress.

Sometimes negative actions and even subconscious feelings, may be the result of a person's desire or need for attention. Some parents are so busy they don't or find it hard to take time to notice a child at all, unless the child draws attention through bad behavior, or unless they are sick. This parenting pattern and others can encourage negativity.

Children can be conditioned by their parenting to diminish and erase themselves and be completely selfless. I was brought up this way, and I know what it's like to be broken open and even knocked down. It took me many years of work to change the resulting negative self-image. Although overcoming the negativity of my upbringing seemed an impossible task at times, I believe I have **succeeded** and become more than I ever thought I would be, and I'm **happy** with myself now.

It's a tragic fact that emotional trauma is often passed down through families, and children inherit their parents' dysfunctions. That's why it's very important to remember that it's not our fault, when our families pass on learned negative experiences. They don't mean to hurt us, but it happens, even in the most **loving** families.

Just being a woman, can make us more susceptible to negativity, according to relationship expert Dr. John Gray, who says women tend to be more negative than men. I think one reason is because of programming from fashion magazines and TV ads, leaving us feeling insecure over the tiniest flaw. Their air-brushed images often send the message, whether intentional or not, that we're not good enough.

We don't always decide to be negative. Even if we have a positive childhood experience, something tragic can happen to us or to those we love, or we suffer extended periods of physical or emotional abuse after childhood. It's only normal to react with sadness, anger, distrust or fear to these extreme situations.

Sometimes those who suffer these tragedies or other trauma don't have the time to grieve or heal, before they're hit with another unhappy or stressful event.

Therefore, they stay stuck with feelings from the past that become even more pronounced and powerful— sometimes moving into depression, hatred, cynicism and hostility. By then, they are so used to seeing the negative side of life, they become stuck in that mindset and understandably so.

As a result, they start to act out, negatively, and then feel bad because of their behavior. It can turn into a seemingly endless cycle—one that can lead to constantly bringing others down, in an attempt to make themselves feel better. They never compliment anyone. They think in extremes; everything is always black or white—forgetting about gray. They can even become abusive themselves.

It is only natural for others to respond to this negativity, in a way that increases and reinforces it. It's no wonder, then, that those who are negative, suffer from loneliness and low self-esteem, and they yearn for something to make them feel cared about and acknowledged. It may take some kind of jolt or awakening to help them realize that their thoughts, still stuck in the past, are controlling the way they feel and the way they act now.

A rather new and interesting theory that answers the question of "why am I negative," comes from Rick Hanson, Ph.D., a neuropsychologist, a best-selling author and founder of the Wellspring Institute for Neuroscience and Contemplative Wisdom.

Hanson says that, because of early survival instincts that alerted us to danger signals, humans are evolutionarily wired to have a negative bias. That's because it was more important for our earliest ancestors to avoid threats than it was to collect rewards.

Therefore, our modern minds evolved, with a natural tendency to discard the good and focus on the bad. So, while the amygdala in our brains easily stores negative information, as a survival mechanism, we have to hold positive thoughts much longer, for them to be stored in our long-term memories. This is why it takes a little more work, practice and repetition, to help us move from a negative to a more positive focus on life.

Finally, stress may have more impact on the way we think, act and look, than any other factor. We will discuss stress, its impact and ways to alleviate it more fully, under the "SOLUTIONS" and other sections in this book.

There are many different aspects to having a tendency toward negativity. Sometimes there are physical causes, like traumatic brain injury, hormonal imbalances, post-traumatic stress disorder and others, which we will also discuss more fully and offer treatment suggestions for these conditions. Whatever the cause of the negativity, we will take a closer look at several of them and discuss various ways, to help you **overcome** and **break free** of these issues that plague you.

CHAPTER 4

BENEFITS OF OVERCOMING NEGATIVITY

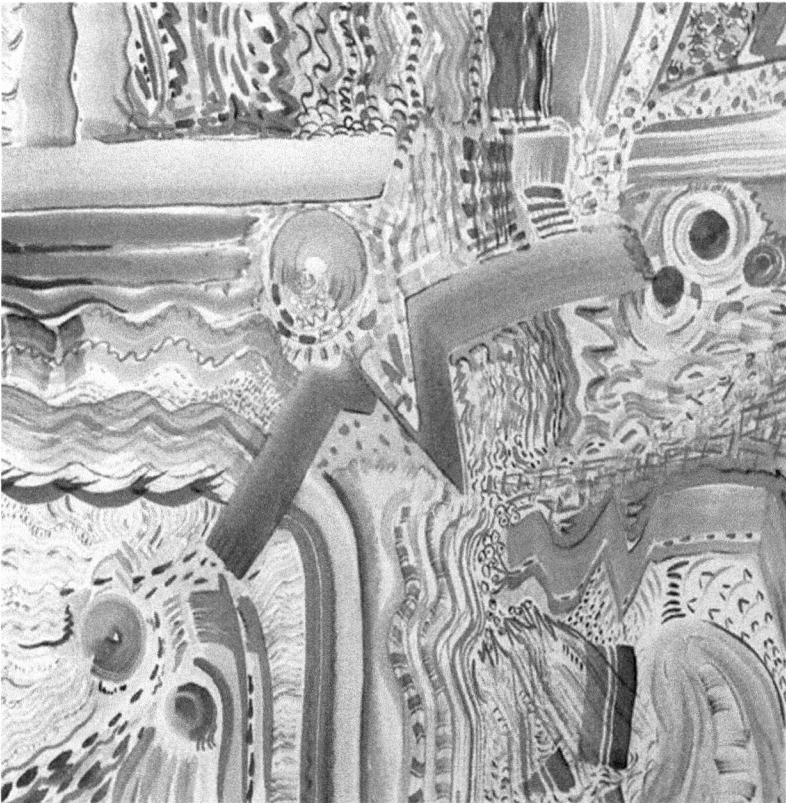

Henry Brown

"Letting go of and overcoming negativity will give you
More control over your personal growth and
confidence.

— Vivian Orgel

WHY CHANGE?

While change is a **new beginning**, new beginnings don't have to be scary. If you're happy with your career, your relationships, your health and your life, in general, then maybe you don't need to change. However, if there are aspects of your life you'd like to **improve**, either minor or major ones, you'll find that moving out of a negative mindset can be the key to **success**. After all, how can you enjoy life if you always look at everything negatively? If you do, you must consider that you might be addicted to this way of thinking.

On the **up side**, lifting our minds out of negativity can be a **wonderful**, **transforming** and even **exuberant** experience. We can actually feel positivity, emotionally and physically—revealing how **beautiful** we can really be.

Ridding ourselves of negativity, can show through our skin and body. Becoming more positive, can allow us to be more **charismatic**. As a result, making **friends** and keeping them will become much easier.

Negative thinking can taint your relationships with others, and it can discolor your perception of yourself and your worthiness. Placing limitations on your worthiness, not only decreases your self-esteem, but it can also cause a ripple of problems in many other areas of your life.

Changing your mindset, can help remove these negative tides of change. It will give you a **fresh** perspective on life. The way we choose to think about the past or certain things that happen in our lives, can have a huge impact on just about everything. It can even drain us of the energy we need to get through the day.

However, did you know that altering your perspective, can give you the **energy** you need and **desire** or that having a positive attitude and **believing** in yourself, can actually **improve** your auto-immune system?

Overcoming negativity, has many significant health benefits.

These Include:

• 	Increased life span

• 	Lower rates of depression

• 	Lower levels of distress

• 	Greater resistance to the common cold — or an **enhanced** immune system

• 	Better overall psychological and physical **well-being**

• 	Reduced risk of death, from cardiovascular disease.

• 	Resistance to digestive diseases/conditions

- Better ability to **cope** with stress

- **Improved** sleep

- Enhanced feelings of self-worth

- Greater **confidence**

- More **resilience**

- Greater success—goal **achievement**

How we process, manage and direct negative emotions, impacts us physically, as well as emotionally. Those who frequently feel these negative emotions may experience subconscious muscle clenching, which can cause extreme tension which, in turn, can affect not only how we feel, but how we look, showing up as skin wrinkles, for example (lip line, forehead creases, etc.).

These same emotional responses tax the adrenal glands. Anger does this, by keeping the body on constant alert, not giving it time to repair itself. This leads to the breaking down of the skin's elasticity and collagen, which advances sagging. This can happen anywhere in the body, in addition to tensing body muscles.

Smiling, happy people are naturally more **attractive** to others. Below are beauty benefits to overcoming negativity, some mentioned above and more:

- Clearer, healthier skin

- Fewer or no wrinkles

- Less skin sagging

- Higher levels of skin hydration

- More **active** genes associated with youth

When negative emotions are left unchecked and untreated for long periods of time, the risk of hypertension, cardiovascular disease, digestive diseases and infection becomes much greater. If it reaches a point that it impairs the entire immune system, any part of the body can be adversely affected. It can even give you a slew of sexual problems.

Have you ever been unable to perform for your partner? It may be because you're too stressed out from dealing with so many negative thoughts and emotions.

Even nervous excitement can negatively impact the body. Tension management first requires awareness. Then it's important to use the energy from emotions as a source of motivation, to get necessary things done and divert harmful consequences, such as premature aging and burnout.

Calming down is only one preventive measure.

Reeducating ourselves to perceive circumstances or life, as a whole, differently, can help us **manage** our emotions better. Any **improvement** is a step toward feeling better and looking better.

Essentially, positive thinking can greatly **enhance** our physical, as well as, our emotional well-being. You *can* begin to cut through problems and learn solutions to restore your emotional balance. If you decide to change your way of thinking, you will learn, through tips in this book and other ways, to redirect and recondition yourself, to get beyond negative thoughts and beliefs. Life offers many challenges, but we can learn to get through the hurt, the broken promises, the heartbreaks and the setbacks.

Without challenges, we don't grow. We can learn and earn, but it's not going to give us the depth we experience through challenges. So, don't be afraid of them; grow and go through them.

We *can* train our brains to think **forward,** instead of staying depressed and remaining where we are. Even the slightest attitude adjustment, can lead us to longer, healthier and happier lives.

EFFECTS OF NEGATIVE THINKING ON THE BRAIN

We now know that brain injury or damage can cause us to become abnormally consumed with negative thoughts, feelings and actions, which can make overcoming negativity more difficult than it is for others, not so injured. But we also learn, from recent research, that getting stuck on negative thoughts, alone, can actually result in physical damage to the brain. Continually turning a situation over and over in the mind, focusing only on its negative aspects, or "ruminating," can actually damage the neural structures in the brain that regulate feelings, emotions and memory, according to Andrew Newberg, M.D, a pioneer in the field of neurotheology.

Newberg and co-author Mark Waldman write about **fascinating** new research that reveals the effect that just seeing or hearing negative words can have on the brain.

Newberg explains that, if you were put into an MRI scanner (a device that takes a video of your brain), and the word "NO" was flashed in front of your eyes for less than even a second, the picture your brain would produce would show "a sudden release of dozens of stress-producing hormones and neurotransmitters," chemicals that would "immediately interrupt the normal **functioning** of your brain, impairing logic, reason, language processing, and **communication**."

Seeing a list of negative words for just a few seconds, says Newberg, can have an even greater impact. They have the power to make an anxious or depressed person feel worse, and the more you focus on them, the more disruptive these words can be, even to the point of disrupting your life and affecting sleep, appetite, and your ability to experience long-term joy and satisfaction.

Vocalizing, on top of seeing the word, "No," adds Newberg, increases the effects on your brain even more, and not just your brain, but the listener's brain as well. Thus parents, teachers and other authority figures can have a profound effect upon children, just by the way they teach them to behave or learn. Most important, says Newberg, "if you teach them to **think positive,** you can turn their lives around."

Further research on the effects of negative thinking on the brain, is even more revealing. As noted earlier, there is now scientific understanding that humans have evolved to focus on the negative, as a mechanism necessary for **survival**. As humans, we learned, during our first years on earth, how to respond quickly to serious safety threats. However now, when we worry or have negative thoughts over issues that are not life-threatening, our brains don't know the difference and are tricked into thinking there is an immediate threat, which leads to stress and the fight-or-flight response.

On the other hand, if we train ourselves to think more positively about the challenges we face, then our brain assumes the situation is safe and under control, and it doesn't create the stressful reaction that leads to other negative results.

More specifically, it's the thalamus in our brains that gets confused, when we send negative messages. It doesn't realize that the thoughts are not the same as real danger, so it reacts, by sending motor and sensory signals to the rest of the body, preparing it to flee. This puts us in a state of arousal, which causes us to sweat and breathe harder. That increases our heartbeat and raises our blood pressure and puts us in a state of stress.

We will further discuss the effects that chronic stress can have on our health, our looks and our happiness. If we allow the negative thinking to go on, uninterrupted, the stress that's created can change the brain enough to cause numerous mental or emotional disorders, some as serious as ADHD or others that are considered very serious mental conditions.

What's most important to realize and remember, is that we can interrupt harmful negative thinking, through use of **positive thoughts** and/or actions and prevent the difficult or worst outcomes of our natural tendency to focus on the negative. *We simply must train ourselves to replace negative thoughts with positive ones.*

This is where the suggestions included in this book come in. They help us change the negative "ruminations" that can be self-perpetuating and lead to brain damage, less attractive appearance and more negative outcomes. Newberg tells us that the faster we can interrupt the amygdala's reaction to a negative thought or imagined threat, the more likely we'll reduce the possibility of "burning a permanent negative memory" into our brains. So please consider making good use of the practice examples, within and at the end of this guide to overcoming negativity, to help you become a **pro** at replacing negative thoughts with **positive** ones.

CHAPTER 5

THE POWER OF YES

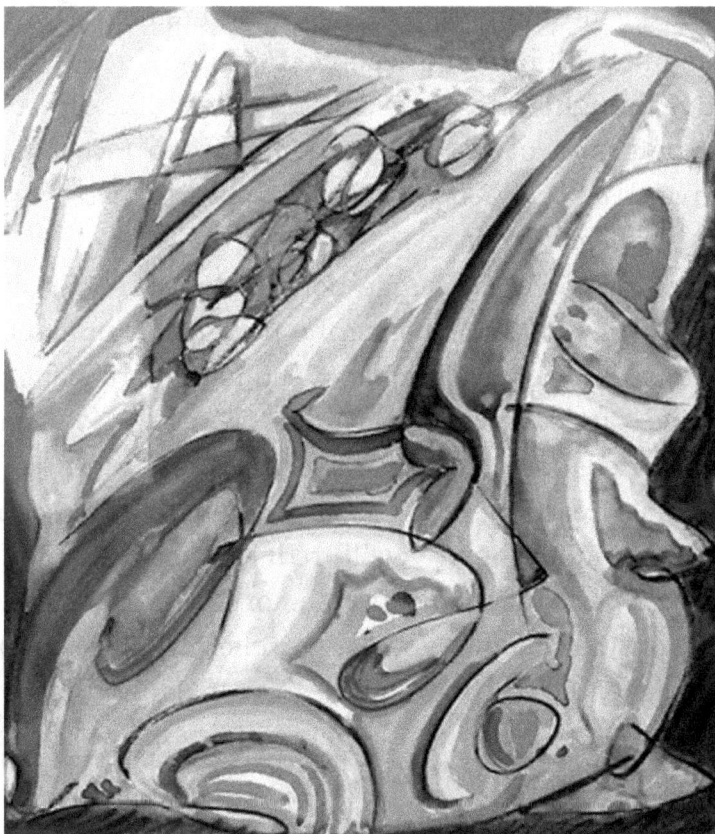

Henry Brown

Yoko Ono won John Lennon's heart with one simple,
but powerful word, "Yes."

If negative thoughts—and even the word, "no"—can
lead to chronic stress and eventually damage the brain and
our lives, in general, imagine what the **Power of Yes** can do.

Now we know that evolution has wired us to pay more attention to the negative, rather than the positive, aspects of a situation. On top of this natural tendency to focus on the negative, some of us, for one reason or another, may have a very difficult time focusing on, or even acknowledging, the **"Yeses"** in our lives.

Some experts say it takes as many as 28 "yeses" (positive thoughts, words or events), to cancel out every "no" we encounter. Others say three "yeses," for every "no," may be enough to burn more positives into our memories.

Whatever it takes, the **up side** of putting forth the effort is that it is **well worth** it. My life is evidence of how the **power** of positive thinking can overcome any obstacle or serious trauma we face. And now science backs up what I have learned in the school of life and have shared with others.

The story of how John Lennon met and fell in **love** with Yoko Ono, can be seen as an allegory for what it takes to get to the "Yes" in our lives and the **reward** for making that effort. As John told the story, he had come to see Yoko's art exhibit at the Indica Gallery in London. One of the exhibits required that the viewer climb a ladder, then pick up an attached magnifying glass, in order to read the tiny word, painted on a canvas attached to the ceiling. The message was simply, "Yes." John later said, in an interview, that he was **"relieved"** that the message was "positive." That is the meeting that sparked their long relationship, said John.

Dr. Rick Hanson, the researcher who publicized the theory of our evolutionary negativity, trains others on how to replace negative thoughts with positive ones, and his reports on the outcomes he sees, from this training, reveal rewards that are **priceless**.

Hanson, I and others have proven that humans can overcome negativity and, as a result, experience significantly less stress and depression and much more **self-esteem, confidence, gratitude** and overall **happiness**. It may take commitment and work, but it's worth it.

And one more thing, once we get a taste of this **happiness** and **peace**, we want more and are motivated to create more **joy** in our lives through the power of YES.

PART II

SOLUTIONS
Steps Leading to "YES"

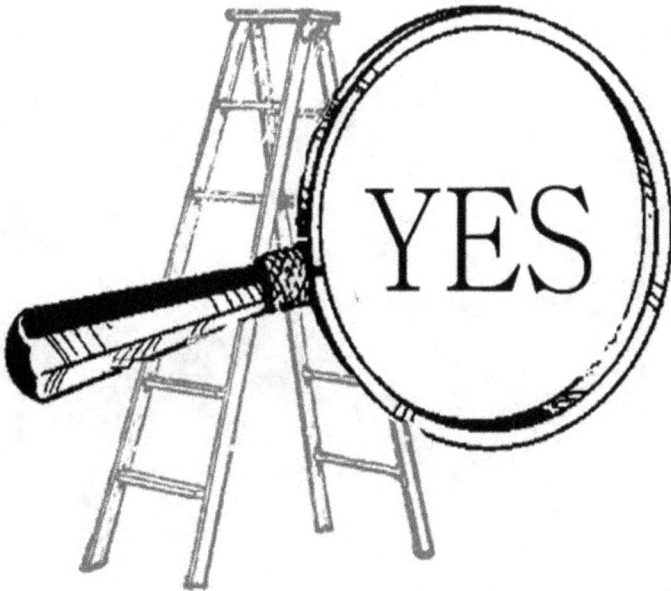

CHAPTER 6

BEGIN THE PROCESS OF CHANGE

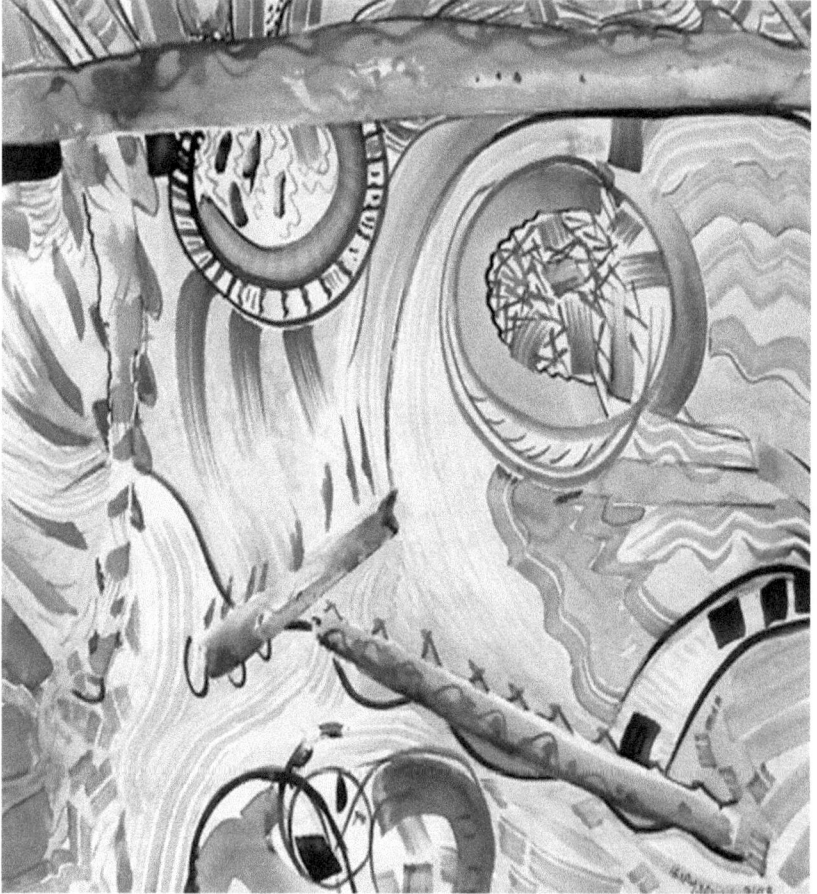

Henry Brown

"Change your thoughts and you change your world."
— Norman Vincent Peale

If you've read this far, you have likely decided you may, or do, need to overcome negativity. Overcoming negativity, begins with **awareness** of the problem. Then, the next step is to change the way we think. We do this, mainly, by **calming** down the negative noise in our minds, then finding replacement thoughts, changing our perspective and our focus, developing **gratitude** and learning to **forgive**.

With these tools, we then become equipped to deal with life's stresses and other obstacles we encounter.

We will suggest many more ways to expand on these basic practices, to make your life more positive. Some of the suggestions will be repeated, because the same ones help us recover from different causes of negative thinking. But basically, they all fit into six major steps we can take to lead us to the top rung of our ladder and tapping more into the power of "Yes."

These steps are:

1. Acknowledge the problem; Deal with denial.

2. Calm your mind.

3. Replace negative with positive.

4. Divert the senses; Embrace beauty.

5. Develop an attitude of gratitude.

6. Forgive yourself and others.

No matter what has caused or led to our current state of negative thinking, the above steps can pull us from out of the mud we're stuck in and onto the ladder, heading upward toward our goals. Maybe more important, is that taking steps to make positive changes in your life, creates more **self-love.**

STEP 1. DEAL WITH DENIAL

"If I think about it now, I'll go crazy. I'll think about it tomorrow."
—Scarlet O'Hara, from Margaret Mitchell's *Gone with the Wind.*

Denial is a thought process we go through, in which we convince ourselves something is not true or not really an issue. However, admitting negative feelings, might be the best way to **release** them.

That said, it's not always easy to be **aware** of our own excessively negative thought patterns—after all, just acknowledging them, itself, seems negative. However, especially now that we know humans are naturally wired to focus on negativity, it's certainly nothing to beat ourselves up over.

In fact, in addition to being an inherited survival mechanism, negativity can also be a coping mechanism. If you can simply deny behaviors, feelings and thoughts, and especially what may have created them, then you don't have to deal with them. Right?

Even though denial is hard to self-realize, if you are thinking, feeling and acting out most of the examples, listed in Chapter 2 and repeated below, you are likely stuck in negativity.

A. Negative Thoughts

- Focusing only on the problem

- Everything bad happens to me

- I can't help it

- Over generalizing (always, never)

- Polarizing (only good or bad)

- Never satisfied

B. Negative Emotions/Feelings

- Jealousy

- Anger/Irritability

- Low self—esteem

- Worthlessness

- Helplessness

- Feeling stuck—in a rut

C. Negative Actions

- Blaming others

- Abusing oneself or others

- Criticizing others, to divert attention from oneself

- Getting and staying stuck in negative patterns or old thinking habits

- Selfishness/self-absorption — It's always about you

- Controlling/manipulative

D. Negative Inaction

• Procrastination or Paralysis —negative thoughts cause us to put off or keep us from doing what needs to be done or achieving our goals.

Although it takes **courage** to face some of life's harsh realities, eventually we have to deal with these issues. In fact, we can find a positive way to deal with them that will work to our advantage.

If I'm upset, I have to put on the brakes and realize that, most of the time, what I was upset about is over—it happened at another time—and it doesn't have to ruin the rest of my day or my life.

Staying in negativity, can stunt your growth and keep you in a rut. However, becoming self-aware, can motivate you to take more control over your life.

Try to keep in mind that there's nothing negative about owning up to negativity and nothing wrong with, giving yourself time to process what has led you to develop negative thinking or, giving yourself time to experience any delayed grief.

Pacing yourself as you take the steps to overcome the past and the negativity that came with it, is perfectly ok, even recommended. But the next step to overcoming negativity and living a happier and fuller life, is getting beyond denial and getting on with a willingness to start actively focusing on the positive aspects of our lives.

If you know the story of Margaret Mitchell's *Gone with the Wind*, you know that, even though Scarlet gives herself a break from dealing with her uncomfortable realities, it doesn't take her long to confront them head on.

STEP 2. CALM YOUR MIND

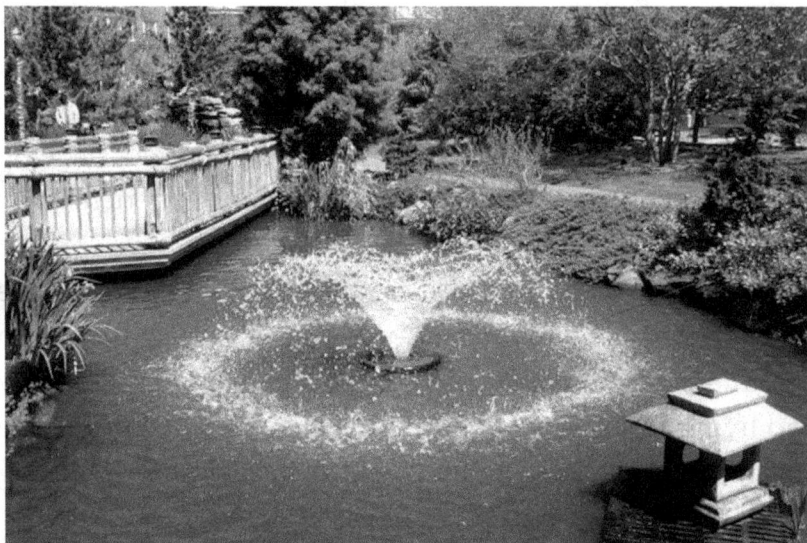

Vivian Orgel

Once a day, or at least several times a week, find somewhere you can go, away from distractions, where you can spend a few moments or more, surrounded by **peace and quiet**, preferably a **belvedere**, a place with a **beautiful** view. To clear your mind and emotions, you can **meditate**, **pray** or just focus on the **peace, quiet and beauty** of your surroundings.

On one of Dr. Phil's recent programs, he sought to help a **pretty** young woman who saw herself as ugly. Her negative self-image was so debilitating, she rarely socialized or even left her home.

Dr. Phil explained to her why it was so important to clear her mind of negative thoughts because, he says, we contain in our minds many times more thoughts than the negative words we speak—words that can, themselves, burn a lasting impression in our brains.

So, before we can begin to work on replacing so many negative thoughts, we need to **calm** down our minds and clear out as much negativity as we can.

For some, simply writing down these thoughts can be a way of clearing them out of their minds, so long as they don't focus on the negatives and eventually move on to positive replacement thoughts. At the end of the book, I provide lined pages for journaling, if you would like to try this one way to help clear your mind of negative thoughts and emotions.

STEP 3. REPLACE NEGATIVE WITH POSITIVE

"Thoughts become things. Choose the good ones."
—Mike Dooley

Our emotions are produced from our thoughts and beliefs. If I think something happening today will be the same as it was in the past, it may seem that way now. So, it's not enough to just clear our minds of negative thoughts; we need to replace the negatives with **positives**. Until we have changed our habit of negative thinking, this may take some work.

Below, I've included some exercises to help you practice, replacing negative thoughts with more positive, **constructive** ones. Use this section to practice, whenever and as often as you feel the need.

EXERCISES ON THOUGHT REPLACEMENT

Below are questions to prompt you to think about your feelings—to help you identify what they are and where they are coming from, with lines for you to write your answers.

Next you are encouraged to write down alternatives. See the example below, to give you an idea of how I'd approach this exercise.

EXAMPLE:
What happened today?
I lost my job.

What am I feeling?
Insecurity, anger, embarrassment

What am I thinking?
I won't find another job.

What else could I think?
I've learned a lot and also what I needed from this job, which is helpful in getting me to where I ultimately want to be in my career.

NOW YOU TRY
• **What have I been doing or what has happened today?**

_____

_____

_____

How do I feel about what happened?

_____

_____

_____

_____

_____

_____

_____

_____

- **What am I thinking?**

_____

_____

_____

_____

_____

- **What else could I think?**

_____

_____

_____

_____

• **How do I feel now?**

_____

_____

_____

_____

_____

_____

_____

_____

_____

_____

Below is one example of how I changed my perspective about a stressful situation. By changing my focus to a positive view of the situation, I am able to alleviate my stress. Instead of fretting over all my unfinished projects, I changed my thinking to: "Even though I have some work left to do, I have already accomplished and completed many things."

MORE ON CHANGING OUR PERSPECTIVE AND FINDING REPLACEMENTS FOR NEGATIVE THOUGHTS

"When you are distressed by an external thing, it's not the thing itself that troubles you, but only your judgment of it. And you can wipe this out at a moment's notice."

—Marcus Aurelius

Let's look at a few more tips on how to tackle negative thinking, by viewing things in a different way.

- Make sure you have accurate information before you size up a situation—before you act or react.

- Be mindful of your feelings about a situation.

- Stop and clearly assess the situation—distance yourself from your emotions and thoughts.

- Learn to distinguish between your feelings and the facts.

- Your feelings can be tainted by the past. Be sure to deal with present.

- Realize that every challenge does not have to be taken so seriously. Some things are just not worth the worry. "Don't sweat the small stuff."

- Pleasing everyone is not required or advisable. When confronted with a question you don't want to answer, give yourself permission to ask, "Why do you want to know?" and permission not to answer at all.

- If the challenge needs to be confronted, welcome it. **Believe** that it can be overcome. **Overcoming** will show how **resilient** you can be.

- Focus on the positive aspects of everything you encounter.

- Stress doesn't have to get the better of you. See it as a **motivator** to **growth**. It can teach you new **answers** and **open up endless possibilities**.

- We all have flaws. Admit them, without dwelling on them. Remind yourself everyday of your **strengths and assets**.

- **Success** and **worth** are not determined by how much money you make.

- See fears only as obstacles, not barricades, in the road to **happiness** and success. We can walk around the obstacles.

- **Believe** in yourself. See all people, including yourself, as **valuable,** with a **unique** story to share and a unique purpose to fulfill. There is **absolutely** no one who can replace you or what you were given to bring to this world.

Now, let's expand on some of these points. First, it's extremely important to have accurate and complete information about a situation, before you decide how to think about it.

Getting upset over something that didn't really happen or a misunderstanding, is a waste of time and **energy**, which can create unnecessary stress, negative feelings—and even worse, negative actions that lead to more problems and stress. So, get the facts, before you react.

Once you have the facts, try to be **mindful** of your feelings. Determine if what you are feeling is based on what is happening now or influenced by things from the past. Try to deal only with what is happening in the present. Also examine the way you see the situation. Ask yourself if it is really 100% negative, and try to find positive angles to what is going on and what it could mean. What has the most impact is *the meaning you attach to the event or thought.*

When real problems arise, try to view them as **opportunities** to **grow**. Realize that if you become resistant or upset, that reinforces the problem and gives it more power over you. Reacting negatively, can overtax your nervous system and deplete the energy you need to **successfully** confront the problem.

Accept that stress is a part of life—it's always there, in everything you do. There would probably be something wrong with you, if you didn't have stress in your life. What's important is how you interpret, **recycle** and use it. Stress can be the **motivator,** to help you **excel** and turn a bad situation into preparation for the future. As you begin to use stress to your advantage, you will be amazed at how **resilient** you can be, and then you can use that **resilience** to gain **confidence and self-worth**, which will make confronting future challenges **easier**.

Make it your mission to clear out unnecessary, repetitive and annoying, self-defeating perceptions. Most important, replace your negative thoughts with something better.

We are learning more every day about how negative thoughts affect the mind and the body. Emotional or mental stress stores in the body and eventually does harm. Wouldn't you be **happier**, if you could use some of these ideas to change a mindset that is putting up roadblocks to your physical and mental **well-being**?

Following are two more examples from my life experience, showing how I was able to Turn Stress Positive.

EXAMPLE #1

Due to a plumber's shoddy work, I endured a huge flood and wound up living in a rental apartment. All the wood floors and carpet had to be ripped out and the air ducts dried; and the walls had to be repainted and furniture removed. The place was unlivable.

However, I kept my **cool**. I reminded myself that I had previously spent eight months dealing with similar conditions (including living out of shopping bags), due to a catastrophic apartment fire. I drew on that experience to take positive actions, instead of focusing on what was wrong. I was determined to **recover** my expenses, which were, at this

54

point, losses. I hired an expert plumber, at the suggestion of the insurance company, to do a report. Then I filed a claim against the other plumber who caused the damage.

Initially, there was a scheduling mix-up by the court clerk, and my plumbing expert was never notified of the court date. I almost lost him, which would have meant losing the case, before even getting started. This could have been completely negative and highly stressful, but I was determined. I put in the time it took to identify the exhibits, got the loan expense reports, copies for the judge, opposing lawyer and myself. I was up against an insurance lawyer. But because I'd been to court many times dealing with bad tenants. I felt that I knew how to handle myself, so I went in on my own.

I use to get nervous, unable to sleep the night before, and made myself miserable (and complained to people close to me). It turned out the fear and anticipation was the worst of it. I soon realized that I was handling things well, even with all the court deadlines.

On the day of the court appearance, I presented my case well and discovered I had all the skills needed. When I interviewed the plumber who was at fault, I came up with some good questions I hadn't thought of before that were helpful to my case.

I derived so many positive benefits from this seemingly negative experience, that I'm now even more confident and proud of myself. I have become a better public speaker, and I don't see myself having the court jitters again, anytime soon.

My newfound coping skills may be put to the test soon. In the state of Virginia, a lawyer is allowed to appeal and move the case to another court. I may have to start over again.

But that's ok. I will focus on what I can learn to further develop my presentation skills, which I will use in my webinars and lectures. I'm ready.

EXAMPLE #2

I sent a story to the webmaster for my blog. Then I updated it. But because I couldn't get it off my phone, I had to rewrite it. I learned a long time ago that, instead of getting upset, I would end up writing a better version. I already knew most of the story, so it would be a piece of cake.

I believe that when things go wrong, you learn from the experience, and that makes dealing with challenges easier, the next time around. As a result, things usually get better.

Remember: While change is a new beginning,
new beginnings don't have to be scary.   .

STEP 4. FIND A DISTRACTION—EMBRACE BEAUTY

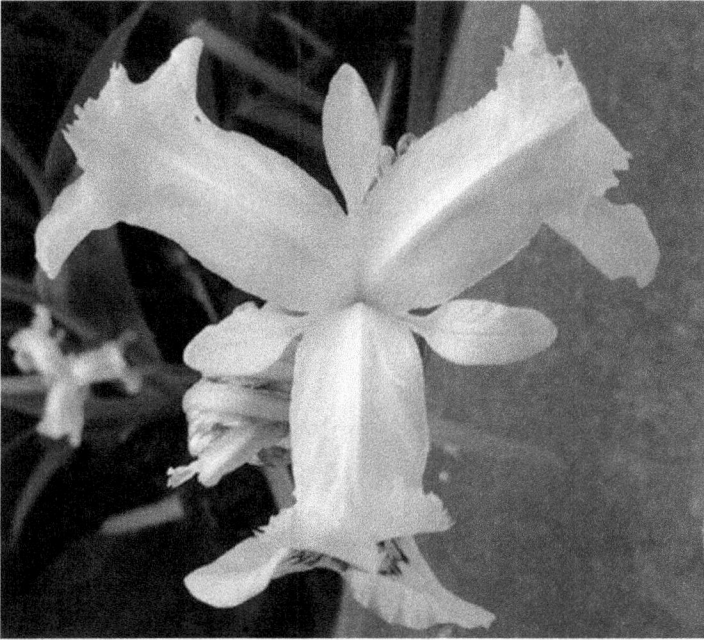

Vivian Orgel

"Everything has beauty, but not everyone sees it."

— Confucius

Find something **peaceful** and/or **pretty** to focus on every day. Diverting attention from your problems and focusing on something of **beauty**, is a **time-honored** method of **improving** or combating stress and negativity. Some find **solace** in a walk in the woods, some in contemplating a **rose** or other thing of natural beauty. A walk through an art gallery or attending a concert in the park, can also be incredibly **soothing** to the soul.

Anything that can make you **smile,** has the power to change your thoughts—something as small as a smile can have a huge impact over the rest of your day and that of others with whom you interact.

Alcoholics Anonymous and Al-Anon's "One day at a Time" is full of anecdotes, quotations and tips that can help change what alcoholics and their loved ones often refer to as "stinkin' thinking." Many of these daily meditations advise readers to contemplate something of beauty, as a way of breaking the spell negative thoughts can have over our feelings and our lives.

When you are focusing only on what's wrong, you're blocking advancement, **opportunities, happiness** and even blocking **love.** Give your focus on pain and stress a **rest,** by **embracing** the **beautiful, peaceful** parts of life. They are there for you to notice.

STEP 5. DEVELOP AN ATTITUDE OF GRATITUDE

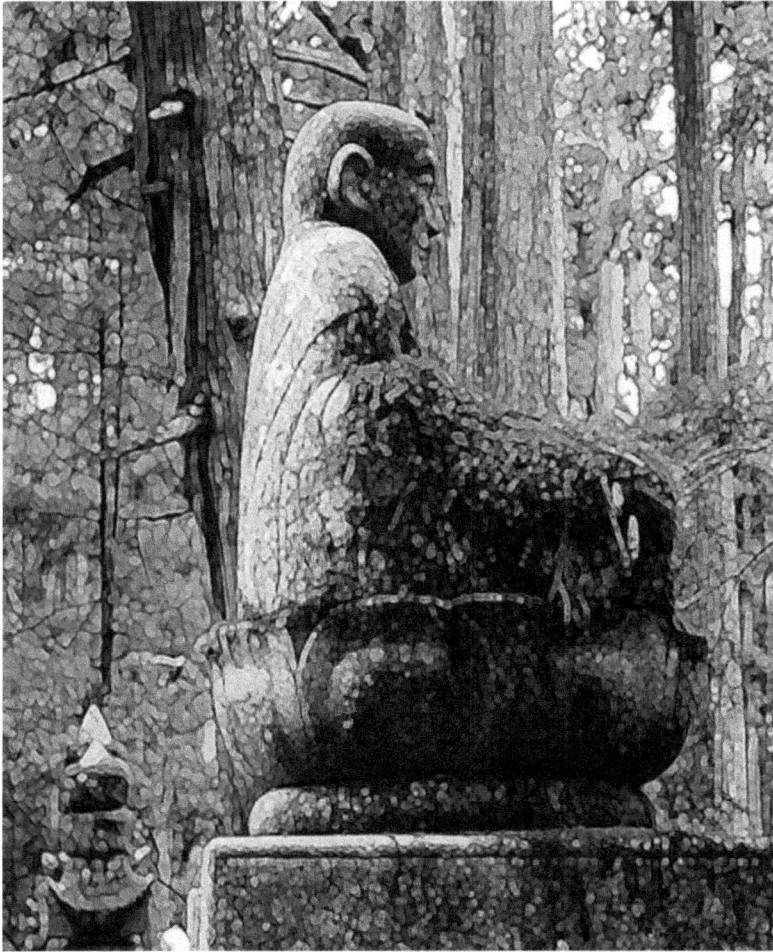

Micah Gampel

"Gratitude is not only the greatest of the virtues, but the
parent of all of the others."   — Cicero

"A noble person is mindful and thankful of the favors he
receives from others."   —The Buddha

You have likely heard it before, but it's worth repeating. It's extremely important to develop an attitude of **gratitude**, and Cicero even considered gratitude to be "the parent of all virtues."

Before studies were done that support what I've been saying for years about the benefits of overcoming negativity, I learned, through experience, how important it is to focus on the positive. That includes being **grateful**, not just for the **special** things that happen or are done for us by others, but for the little things we often take for granted. It all goes along with changing our focus from the bad to the **good**. Now researchers are doing studies to show just how good for you gratitude is. University of California, Davis professor Robert Emmons, considered the world's leading expert on gratitude, found with his research a multitude of physical, psychological and social benefits connected to those who regularly and consistently practice **gratitude**. These include, again, the similar or same ones associated with **positivity**, such as experiencing:

Physical Benefits

- Longer and more **restorative sleep**

- Lower blood pressure

- Improved immune system

- Less noticeable aches and pains

- A tendency to be overall more attentive to health

Social Benefits

- More **empathy** toward others

- A tendency to **forgive**

- A tendency to be helpful and **courteous**

- **Generosity** and **compassion**

- More desire for **social interaction**

- Less loneliness and isolation

Psychological Benefits

- Increased positive emotions

- Feeling of being more **alive, alert** and **awake.**

- Higher levels of **joy and pleasure**

- More **happiness and optimism**

Gratitude helps us recognize and remember that there are **good things** in the world, despite all the bad and ugly that comes with it.

Emmons says **gratitude** is also important, because it shows us a **goodness** that is outside of ourselves—the importance of having "a humble dependence" on others or a higher power. Emmons has developed a list of ways to help us become more grateful.

These include:

- Remembering (but not focusing on) the bad, as a way of helping you recognize the Good.

- Using visual reminders.

- Using words of gratitude, like **"fortunate,"** **"blessed,"** and **"abundance,"**

- Going through the motions to trigger grateful emotions—or as they say in Alcoholics Anonymous, "Fake it, 'til you make it."

- Learning prayers of gratitude or meditating on gratitude.

One of the most effective ways to develop an attitude of gratitude, adds Emmons, is to keep a gratitude journal.

That means setting aside time every day, to actively remind yourself of the **gifts, grace** and other **blessings** you've **enjoyed**. It's also a good idea to find one new thing, every day, that you're grateful for.

As an alternate to journaling, sitting down to write a **thank-you** note can achieve equal results. According to a University of Pennsylvania study, just writing **heart-felt** gratitude notes, alone, can have a profound and lasting effect upon positive thinking. The study discovered that those who composed and sent **sincere** thank-you notes, felt **happier** for weeks after doing so. The same study found that just a week of writing down three positive happenings a day, resulted in months of higher reported **happiness** levels.

More researchers at another university, Eastern Washington, found common positive characteristics among those who express gratitude.
They include:

- **Recognition** of life's small **pleasures.**

- Feelings of **abundance** in their lives.

- **Appreciation** of others' **support of** their **well-being**.

At the end of this book, you will find lined pages for you to start your daily practice of journaling gratitude. Expressing gratitude is important, but there's more. We must show it in some way. There are so many things we can do that will have a positive impact on ourselves and others. Volunteering to read for the sight-impaired or to take a child who doesn't have family out for an afternoon, are just two examples.

As John F. Kennedy once said, "As we express our gratitude, we must never forget that the highest appreciation is not to utter words, but to live by them." Focusing our attention outside of ourselves and helping others, is a very positive way to express our gratitude and increase our own happiness and feelings of **well-being.**

STEP 6. FIND THE PATH TO FORGIVENESS

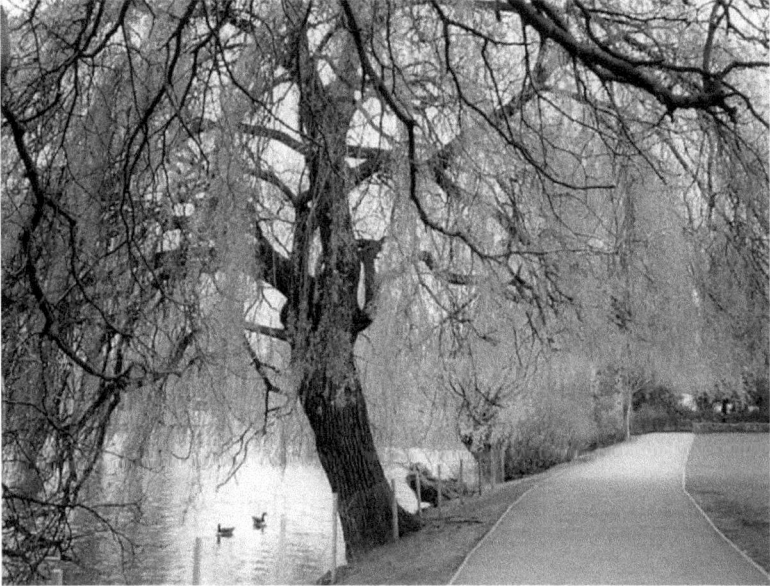

Vivian Orgel

"It's one of the greatest gifts you can give to yourself, to forgive. Forgive everybody." —Maya Angelou

Letting go of grudges from past wrongs, is essential to moving forward and overcoming negativity. According to recent studies, one at Erasmus University, holding a grudge, can literally weigh you down, cause more stress in your life and have a negative effect on your relationships and your health. A Hope College study found that "When people think about their offenders in unforgiving ways, they tend to experience stronger negative emotions and greater stress responses." This is why **forgiveness** is so important to overcoming negative thinking.

In his book on forgiveness he coauthored with his daughter, Archbishop Desmond Tutu explains about the **benefits** of **forgiveness,** to the forgiven, and, especially, to the one who forgives.

Like me, Tutu grew up in an abusive environment, and he says he **understands** how difficult it can be to forgive, He agrees with me and other experts that past traumas we've experienced "live on in our memories," causing new pain in the present and future, as those memories are recalled.

However, he says, the pain we suffer from those memories is only compounded by an "unforgiving heart," and that we always pay a price, if we refuse to forgive. It's not just we who suffer from this refusal. It affects everyone around us—our families, our friends, our communities and ultimately, our entire world, says Tutu, because we are all connected. No one hurts another without having been a victim themselves, and no one is undeserving of forgiveness.To treat anyone less than human, no matter what they have done, he adds, is to participate in the shredding of "the web of **connectedness**," and to suffer consequences from which we cannot escape.

That said, Tutu also explains that forgiveness doesn't mean forgetting or sugar-coating the wrongs that were done to us. He emphasizes that, although it's *not* okay to be abused or injured, violated or betrayed, it *is* okay to forgive. We also must learn to forgive ourselves. Because when we don't let go of the pain or guilt from our past, we continue to punish or torture ourselves. Tutu explains that even though he was just a child, when he witnessed his drunken father abuse his gentle mother, he later felt guilty that he didn't protect her.

Then that guilt turned into self-anger. He was only able to forgive himself, once he was able to no longer hold his father's offenses against him. As a result, he says, those painful memories no longer control his disposition or mood. Forgiveness **liberated** him from a past that had defined him for years.

We forgive, because it is in accordance with the law of our **humanity**, and it is a way to bring **healing** and **peace** to ourselves, says Tutu. He explains that, in his language, one asks for forgiveness by saying "Ndicel' uxolo," which means, "I ask for **peace**." He concludes, emphasizing that "the only way to experience permanent healing and peace," from a wrong done to you or someone you love, is to forgive. Forgiveness is undoubtedly a key aspect of positivity, just as it is with overcoming negative thinking.

Forgiveness Can Also Lead To:

- Improved relationships.

- Lower blood pressure and improved cardiovascular health.

- Decreased risk of diabetes.

- Greater **spiritual** and psychological **well-being**.

- Less anxiety, stress and hostility.

- **Improved** sleep.

- Decreased pain.

- A **stronger** immune system.

- Improved **self-esteem.**

An article on **healthy** aging, by John Hopkins Medicine, agrees that our health depends on **forgiveness**, and that unresolved conflict can go very deep—to the point of damaging our physical, not just our emotional, health. Forgiveness can be as simple as making a choice to let go of the anger and hostility—all the negative feelings—for the person who wronged you, even if they don't deserve it. As you begin to release these feelings of resentment and anger, explains Karen Swartz, an MD who works with mood disorders, you may begin to feel **compassion** and even **empathy** for those who harmed you.

Studies show that the more forgiving people are, the **happier** they are. Johns Hopkins agrees with what I include in these pages and have shared with others for years, that even those who have a hard time forgiving—people stuck in depression and negativity—can learn to think and act in **healthier** ways.

Other experts insist that **cultivating** forgiveness, leads to increased **optimistic** thinking that blocks out negative thinking and also leads to **closer** relationships.

Tutu believes that "The only way to experience permanent **healing** and **peace** is to forgive."

If you'd like to learn more about Tutu's strategy for forgiveness, his book is titled, *The Book of Forgiving: The Fourfold Path for Healing Ourselves and Our World.*

GIVE UP GUILT

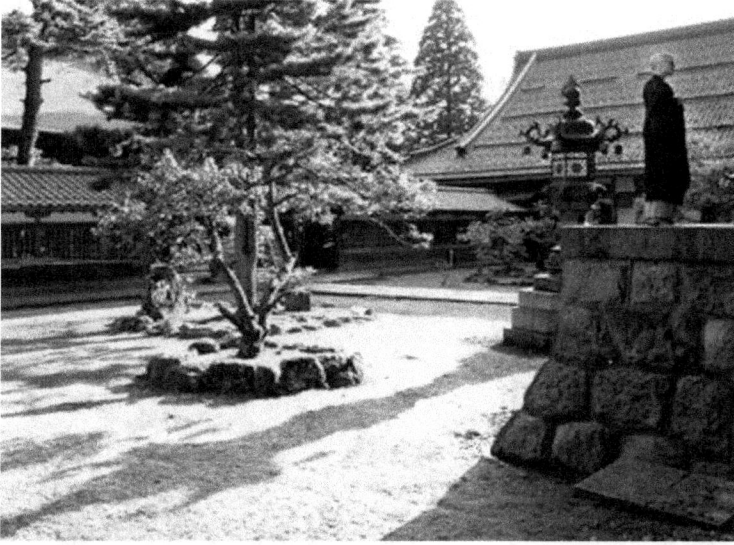

Micah Gampel

A big and essential part of forgiving, is forgiving yourself. You will find that you will repeat past behaviors, especially during your journey to **conquer** negativity. But when you do, be **patient** with yourself. Ask yourself, "Am I burdening myself with guilt?" "Can I forgive myself for making mistakes?"

Know that you can apologize for rude or bad behavior, without beating yourself up. Just do it, and then let it go. And if you are able, make **amends**. Then Stop the mental self-abuse. No one is perfect. Learn how to get rid of the guilt, and you will be more able to acknowledge what you need to work on to improve your life.

CHAPTER 7

MORE ON HOW TO MOVE FROM NO TO YES

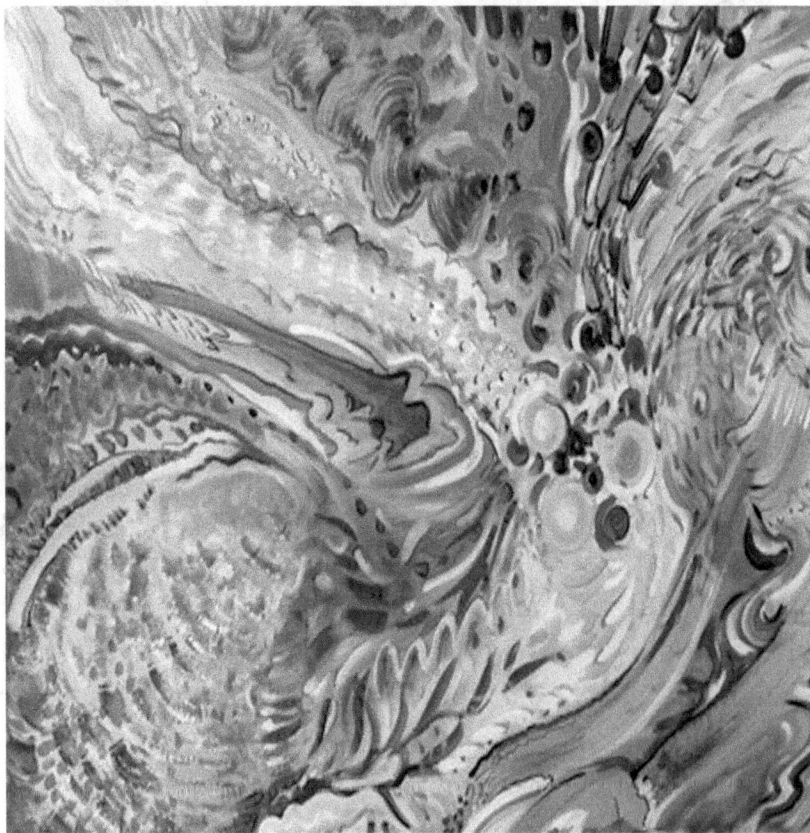

Henry Brown

"Your brain—every brain—is a work in progress. It is 'plastic'."
— Michael Merzenich, Ph.D

PRACTICE AND REPETITION—YES WORDS

We've learned about the **power** of the word, **"Yes"** — much more so, if it's repeated. We've learned that the brain doesn't take our **positive** words and thoughts as seriously as it does the negative ones, simply because it doesn't see them as a threat to our survival.

So, this is where repetition comes in. It is not enough to just think positively, we must be willing to practice consciously generating as many positive thoughts as we can. As noted earlier, it may take as many as 20 or more positives, to cancel out one negative, but three seems to be the minimum, based on what one of the founders of Positive Psychology, Barbara Fredrickson, has discovered.

Fredrickson and her colleagues go on to insist that we must take it a step further and come up with at least five positives, for every negative expression, if we want our business and personal relationships to flourish. A negative expression can be a frown or other negative body language, not just a verbal utterance.

What's really **good news,** is that even if the positive expressions you generate aren't rational, they still have the power to **create** and **enhance** a sense of well-being, **satisfaction** and joy! So, we *can* actually "fake it, 'til we make it."

And don't just engage in positive self-talk, but also share your **happy** and **successful** events with others, which will **reinforce** the positive effects on your brain. We are **encouraged** to **savor**, in every way we can, every positive experience in our lives.

Experts in positive psychology also advise us to speak slowly and choose our words **wisely**; the same advice is given to develop our sense of **gratitude**. Doing so helps to interrupt the brain's tendency to be negative.

More recent research has discovered that simply repeating words like **peace, love** and **compassion.** has the power to activate specific genes that are capable of lowering stress levels.

Repetition is the switch that turns on the power of YES. Feel free to use the alphabet pages at the end of the book, to help you generate at least five positive words for every (or almost every) letter of the alphabet and for every negative thought you find, when you look back over your daily journal. You may also want to pull out the pages and post them around your living or work space as reminders. Another recommended source for **overcoming** the effects of negative expression, is Newberg & Waldman's book, *Words Can Change Your Brain*. Also, you can use the examples of positive self-talk, below, as another way of promoting passive change to negative thought patterns and actions or addictive behaviors, like smoking. Just place **empowering** notes anywhere you are likely to see them often—on light switches, on the fridge, your coffee cup, alarm clock or with your car keys, for example. Leave notes everywhere, especially during stressful times, when you need extra **support**.

Examples of Notes You Can Post for Yourself

- Criticizing myself will not help.

- I will allow myself the sleep I **deserve**—deep, emotionally and physically **restful** sleep.

- It will get done. **Relax**!

Other Motivational Phrases That Are Worth Repeating

- It only takes 30 days, to reprogram new behaviors.

- I'm on my way!

- I will remember to relax.

- A **breakthrough** is inevitable.

- Yes, I can.

- I can use the **energy** from stress, to get things done.

- FEAR stands for "False Evidence Appearing Real."

"Refuse to be average. Let your heart soar as high as it will."

— Aiden Wilson Tozer

PART III

SELF-AWARENESS STRESS AND THE MIND-BODY CONNECTION

"The mind moves the body, and the body follows the mind. Logically then, negative thought patterns harm not only the mind but also the body. What we actually do builds up to affect the subconscious mind and in turn affects the conscious mind and all reactions."
— H.E. Davey, *Japanese Yoga: The Way of Dynamic Meditation*

CHAPTER 8

FROM STRESSING TO BLESSING

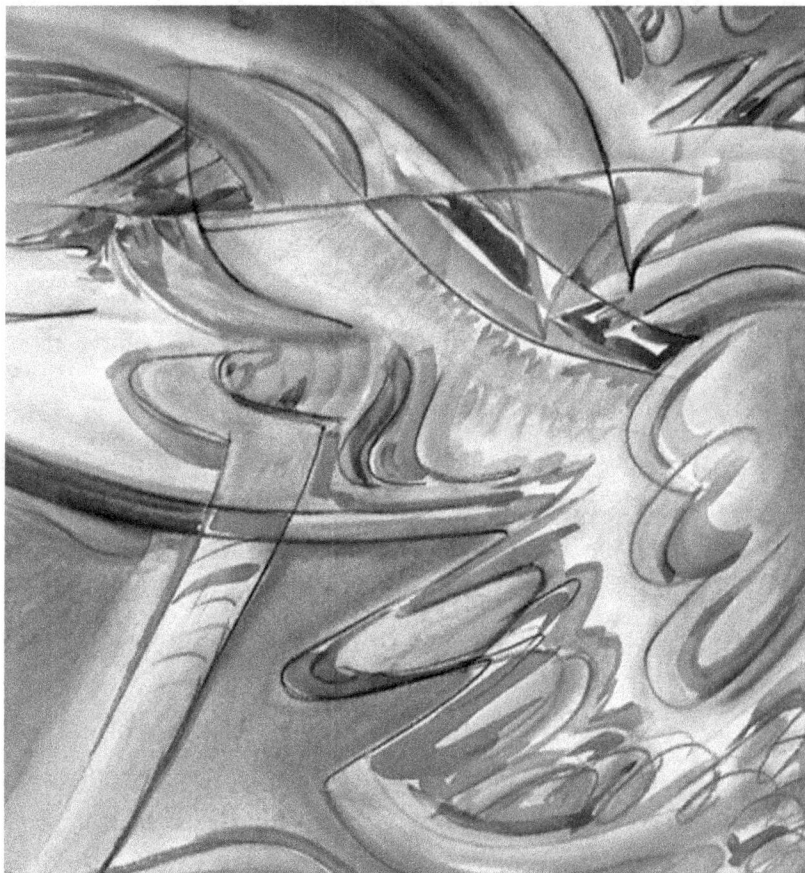

Henry Brown

"The greatest weapon against stress is our ability to choose
one thought over another."

—William James

Self-awareness is the key to set you **free**—the **catalyst** that sets things reacting. Media psychology adjunct professor Linda Durnell writes a blog about the mind-body connection and the effects of stress on our bodies. She says: "When our mind is fearful, our bodies follow the fear, and we experience the physical effects of stress."

You may have heard that stress produces cortisol, the "fat hormone." We know that stress changes our bodily functions and, when left unchecked, can harm us is many ways.

We have felt our body changing when we're asked to do something that we're not ready to do, don't want to do or are expected to do under an imposing deadline.

I know, from my experience and research, that there's a mind-body connection effect to this kind of stress. Think about it. How many of you have gone straight for the bathroom, when you get overwhelmed after a thought? How many of you are lying and don't want others to know? We've all been there. Do you remember in public school, when you had to give a book report or other oral presentation before the class?

I've been aware of the mind-body symptom effect since my early twenties. Sometimes it's not that apparent, but if you look a little bit deeper, you'll find there might be an emotional component to why a person isn't feeling well. A physician client, of mine, called once to reschedule his appointment, saying he had the flu and felt very sick. I asked him when it was that he began feeling what seemed like flu symptoms. In the course of casual conversation, he brought up a car accident that he had testified about in court.

He was found guilty, because he didn't know about a law that says you're not allowed to pass a public bus in the state of Virginia. He suddenly realized that was when he began feeling sick!

Stress *can* cause physical symptoms. It can take a toll on the immune system and leave the body vulnerable to any physical illness. The next time you feel sick, be aware that stress could be the underlying cause.

We must accept that stress is a part of **life**. As long as we're alive, we can't avoid it, but we can **learn optimal** ways to deal with it, so that it doesn't have such devastating effects on all aspects of our lives.

PUT STRESS IN ITS PLACE

Although stress can be a **motivator,** too much of it can seem a formidable roadblock to overcoming negativity. The most effective techniques I can suggest for **relieving** stress, are distraction and exercise. Distraction techniques are believed to be highly **effective** and include using aromatherapy (with **natural** and naturally derived scents like lavender, bay leaves and rose) and using sounds and visual pictures that are found to be effective in pain and mind control.

The idea is to move your mind's attention away from negative stress and toward something more **pleasurable** and immediate. This includes our earlier suggestions to change your focus and try to take time to concentrate on or experience something **soothing** or **beautiful**.

Using the distraction technique, is also good for your physical appearance, because it prevents the stress from settling too deeply into the body and muscles and helps stop the deepening or reinforcement of expression lines.

For physical pain management, one **dependable** distraction technique is to apply pressure to the skin by gently twisting or squeezing the tip of your nose. This works, because pain cannot be felt, at the same level, in two places at the same time. When receiving a shot from a physician or having a bikini wax for the first time, try this technique. Also, changing your posture so you're leaning to one side or leaning forward—or focusing on **relaxing** your shoulders and neck—can distract or inhibit physical sensations. Something else I find helpful, is to lie on your side and move forward and back, as if you're rocking like a baby in a cradle. Movement of any type, can be **helpful**, but because you're lying on your side, it can physically distract your mind—and your pain.

Another distraction strategy involves, redirecting the mind from negative thinking to **productivity**. The goal is to decrease stress and increase **confidence,** by putting **manageable** tasks between seemingly impossible ones. **Conquering** smaller hurdles, makes larger ones seem **easier** to complete. For example, I have redirected my mind to something that **motivates** me, rather than feel a negative emotion. I used the energy from anger, to achieve a better outcome—a good workout from swimming, for example. A third helpful distraction strategy, discussed earlier, works by redirecting your mind away from unpleasant or troubling thoughts, by **engaging** the senses—any or all of them—sight, hearing, touch, smell and taste. It is like turning a channel on the radio or TV, leaving a room to go elsewhere, or just taking a break from what you're currently doing.

Examples include, cuddling or **playing** with a pet, eating something you **like**, watching a child playing or listening to music. (Do choose **music** that doesn't reinforce negative thoughts or emotions).

Your emotions can also be diverted from burdening your mind and body, simply by changing the lighting or temperature—or by exercising.

Yoga is considered to be one of the best exercises for stress. One that particularly promotes **relaxation** and deep breathing, is known as trauma-sensitive yoga, A list of trauma-sensitive yoga instructors, certified by the Trauma Center at the Justice Resource Institute of Brookline, Massachusetts, is found at the link below, listed by country. http://www.traumasensitiveyoga.com/find-a-facilitator.html

By learning and trying these methods, you will find that you can intentionally redirect your mind to control habits, eliminate pressures, decrease anxiety and pain, and improve physical illnesses and skin reactions and conditions. You can move to other tasks, thoughts or mind frames and, therefore, from pain to **peace**. We will discuss more ways to deal with stress, without using drugs. In the meantime:

Don't get stuck in your emotions or make today's story the one that happened in the past!

MORE ON MANAGING STRESS

Managing stress is an essential tool for **overcoming** negativity. We know from Dr. Amen's research, and that of others studying brain damage, that brain health can affect how we think.

And stress, over time, can damage the brain, just as a physical injury can. **Positive thinking** comes more easily, when we deal with and **alleviate** stress, before it builds to a breaking point.

As noted earlier, stress can be a positive, **motivating** force, but sometimes it can be overbearing—piled up bills— the commute to work—difficult relationships, etc. can become overwhelming and affect us in negative ways. During these times, it's important to take **care** of yourself. Most of us are already aware of the importance of the following tips, and we've discussed several already. But when you feel overwhelmed by stress, you still may need to be reminded to:

- **Lighten up** and **Let go.**

- **Exercise—Get Active.**

- **Believe.**

- **Let good things into your life.**

- Breathe deeply—consider yoga as exercise.

- Remember to **laugh**—watch a **funny** film or go see a comedy act.

- Find something of **beauty** to focus on, for at least a few minutes every day.

- Get enough **sleep and rest**.

- Eat **properly** and healthily.

- Talk to someone you **trust**.

- Journal.

- Consider therapy like hypnosis, EMDR and others.

- Build Self-Esteem.

LET GO

Letting go of the past is necessary to keep it from affecting the present and the future. It's important not to get stuck in the emotions surrounding the story you tell yourself that already happened. Don't let the past decide the present or the future, and then don't sweat the small stuff! We do not have to give all of our attention to things that are not priorities, are out of our control or not even a real problem in the first place.

First, as I emphasize earlier, get all the facts about a situation, before you decide whether it's **worth** even confronting. Then decide if there's anything you can do about it. Have you ever heard of the **Serenity** Prayer, asking for help in changing what you can, **accepting** what you can't change and for the "**wisdom** to know the difference?" Many find this prayer or other similar meditations helpful.

Also, we often find that things have a way of working themselves out. We should not let those or ones we cannot control create unnecessary stress. With the numerous life changes that I have endured, I have become **aware** that I don't have to let myself get upset, when things don't go my way.

I was in an exercise class a while back, and about ten minutes before it was over, I noticed on my finger the ring that had just had the diamond reset—a very **special** one I hadn't worn in over two years. It's an **exceptionally beautiful** ring that was passed on through my family. But after the class ended, I saw that the diamond was missing! I began frantically searching everywhere—all over the floor—

looking from a ton of different angles. Still unable to find it, I had to accept that it was lost.

I informed the cleaner at the gym, just in case, and then I left, because I had other pressing matters to take care of. However, once I was no longer busy and had time to think about it, my sadness over the loss of this **precious** keepsake sank in.

The next day I went back to the gym, took out my duffle bag from the locker, and brought it home with me. The zipper was open just a few inches, so I turned it over just to see if there was even the slightest possibility that the diamond had fallen into my bag. When I didn't find it, I put everything back and away, again resigned to having to accept my loss.

But then I found the diamond without trying. On my way to the bathroom in the middle of the night, I stepped on it. The moral of the story is that you never know what's **possible** or how things are going to show up, or when they'll show up for that matter. It's a **good idea** to just be able to let go of things that are out of your control.

GET ACTIVE

"In times of great stress or adversity, it's always best to keep busy, to plow your anger and your energy into something positive."   — Lee Iacocca

In my personal experience, I have found that being **productive** helps decrease the stress effect. If you are **proactive** or have a **doable** list with some available end-points you can quickly **accomplish**, you will feel better about what is happening, if you begin doing these, instead of holding on to the stress and feeling its effects.

I am always busy **becoming** Vivian. One thing I'm good at is keeping busy. I have come to **value** this tool. I use it to distract myself from my emotions. Getting involved in a new project or something that focuses my attention away from my past hurts and trauma, has been the **solution** for me to **overcome** almost anything. Many self-help books suggest being in the moment; I guess this is how I take charge and don't feel vulnerable or victimized.

Why not try something different. Find out what works for you. Instead of complaining, turn your negative thoughts into **productivity**. Learn how to do what was so frustrating to you before.

LIGHTEN UP

Try not to take yourself too seriously or blow isolated incidents out of proportion or take them personally. We can't be perfect; all we can do, much of the time, is admit when we are wrong, apologize and make amends, when possible.

Often when others say or do things that look like a personal attack on us, it really has nothing to do with us; it's all about them. There's often no way for us to know what others are going through in their lives, when they take out their anger or other feelings on us. But if we can decide to withhold judgment of them, it makes it **easier** to be less hard on ourselves. We can all use more **kindness** and **understanding**.

And we, of course, can't control or **fix** everything that happens. Although unfortunate and unfair, sometimes bad, even cruel things, happen to us all. An incident is just an incident—not a time to judge yourself or use as a predictor of the future.

To evaluate how you're doing on the "lighten up" solution ask yourself:

- Am I over-reacting?

- Am I taking myself too seriously?

- How can I be less affected and more *effective*?

BELIEVE

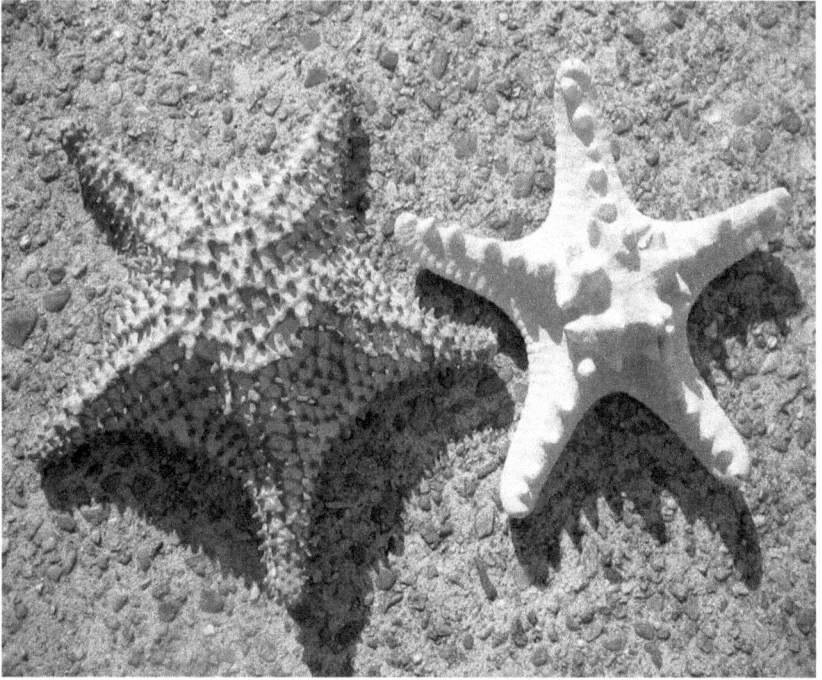

Vivian Orgel

"When your heart is in your dream, no request is too extreme.
When you wish upon a star, your dream comes true."
— Ned Washington & Leigh Harline

Probably the most positive belief you can have is the belief that you **can** change. I have personally **overcome** many catastrophic circumstances in my life and was still able to **transform** them into something **positive**. Although I continue to deal with struggles, I am proof that you, too, can do this. You can overcome negative influences on your life and become a **better** and **happier** person.

I know who I am, and I share this and what I learned with others. My confidence was **earned and deserved**.

If you **believe** in yourself, you can overcome almost anything. Seeing is believing. Just look at other **successful** people in life. Most have overcome many things. In fact, often it was overcoming obstacles that created their success. James Earl Jones overcame stuttering, to become the voice of Darth Vader and CNN. Considered one of the most **effective** and well-known **motivational** speakers ever, Norman Vincent Peale, was once painfully shy and had severe stage fright.

You have to believe that you will overcome anything that is thrown at you, no matter how large or small. One day you will look back and see you have walked miles from the first steps you took to positive thinking. A student once told me, "I knew it was rough, but I wanted to get there; I believed I could."

When you believe in yourself, you believe you can succeed. Success leads to **confidence**, and when you are confident, you realize you **can handle** almost anything that life puts in front of you. So why not **choose** to **succeed** rather than fail? Negativity can bring you down, making everything much harder than it needs to be. It's ok if it doesn't always work out, but **believe** and realize you can **overcome** the outcome, whatever it is.

In her blog about **empowering** and disempowering beliefs, **holistic** nutrition and **fitness** specialist Rhea Morales shares Anthony Robbins' story about the "four-minute mile"—how, for thousands of years, no one believed that a human could run faster, until, in 1954, when Roger Banister broke that negative belief barrier. He succeeded "not merely by physical practice," but "by constantly rehearsing the event in his mind, breaking through the four-minute barrier so many times, with so much emotional intensity that he created **vivid** references that became an unquestioned command to his nervous system to produce the result." Once Banister's **accomplishment** challenged the old belief, others followed in his footsteps.

Morales points out that, today, "Disempowering generalizations about seniors and women are being broken left and right." She concludes her blog, by reminding us that "If we **imagine** success, we will get it. If we imagine failure, that is what we will get. So **free** your mind of any belief that is going to hold you back."

You **CAN** modify the way you think and the way you respond. You can **reboot**—start all over again and do things differently. You have the opportunity for **self-mastery**. You can change your self-talk. You've just gotta put in the time.

LET GOOD THINGS INTO YOUR LIFE

"Joy is what happens to us when we allow ourselves to recognize how good things really are."
— Marianne Williamson

Often negativity leads us to feel we are not worthy or **deserving** of letting **good things** into our lives. These feelings may make it hard for you to ask for what you want. These feelings may be passed on from generation to generation, with parents telling their children, "this is just the way we are," or "this is just the way life is." Comments like "money doesn't grow on trees," or "you're not too old for your wants to hurt you," can become part of your own negative self-talk, negative thoughts, emotions and beliefs that you use on a daily basis to push good things away that might have otherwise easily entered your life.

Fear of rejection or even **pride** (not wanting to look "stupid"), can keep us from asking for what we want and even what we need. Try to see fear as only an obstacle, not a barricade. See the word, "fear," as merely an acronym for "False Evidence Appearing Real," and it will lose some or all of its power over you.

See more about **overcoming** fear in the section on "**Circumventing** Obstacles" and also information about the effects of long-term or traumatic stress, including Post Traumatic Stress Syndrome, and more on effects of negative thinking on the brain. Also, we'll discuss some new and **promising possibilities** for how to treat these, sometimes, disabling conditions.

BUILD SELF-ESTEEM

"One's dignity may be assaulted, vandalized and cruelly mocked, but it can never be taken away unless it is surrendered."
— Michael J. Fox

Much of our **self-esteem** has its roots developed from the past. Eventually we may have to deal with unresolved issues that make us feel bad about ourselves, before we can move on to realizing our **dreams**.

You must earn self-esteem. There is the thinking process and the action itself. Many people find the thinking process helpful. This is where you resolve past issues, **heal** wounds and find the **courage** to like yourself. Self-loathing will seriously undermine progress in all aspects of your life. Some people spend years in this state, where they never reach the point of **acceptance**. Know that the most **important** relationship we will ever have is the one we have with ourselves. Understanding past influences and recognizing past failures, does not mean we have to focus on them. Choose instead to focus on your **strengths**, rather than your faults. You can be **aware** of areas in which you need improvement, without seeing that reality as negative. It just is what it is. Realize that admitting to a weakness, is **strength,** in itself. Put that critical voice to sleep! Thoughts about self-doubt will only hold you back. Try to recognize when you engage in negative self-talk, and stop it before it gets out of hand. Even if you are thinking thoughts like: "This will take forever," or "I'll never be able to do that," try to stop yourself from voicing negative words that reinforce those negative thoughts. Instead of *echoing* the "I can't" thought, take away its power by *saying,* **"I can!"**

Happiness is not **self-esteem**, but it can come with building self-esteem and watching your **personal growth.** As noted earlier, stress can teach us to look for new **solutions**

to problems. It can **motivate** us to **grow**. In turning negatives like stress and fear into positives, we can build self-esteem through these **achievements**, finding **pride** in our positive reactions and actions. Sometimes the deepest wounds prepare us to grow **stronger** and **healthier**. So, **persist**. Make these changes **possible** and **live fully**!

REMEMBER

1.   Low self-esteem hinders us from reaching our goals. We end up tripping over our own feet.

2.   You can learn how to jump-start your success level and get out of the recurring trap you're stuck in.

3.   **Confidence** is the key to relationships, success and decision-making, but wanting confidence and feeling it, are not the same thing. You have to train yourself to live up to your potential.

4.   The past doesn't have to determine the future. Don't get stuck in your emotions and in the story you tell yourself that already happened.

5.   A trigger may only be something you gave too much attention to in the past, maybe an unresolved problem. Don't reinforce it, by giving it power over you, robbing moments better spent otherwise.

"To establish true self-esteem, we must concentrate on our successes and forget about the failures and the negatives in our lives."

— Denis Waitley

"Confidence is not, 'They will like me'. Confidence instead is, 'I'll be fine if they don't.'"

— Christina Grimmie

SOLUTIONS TO DE-STRESS

So, what else can be done to reduce stress? It seems that **relaxed**, **calm** individuals cope with stress differently than tense, aggressive people. The former recognize tension for what it is, and then they try to **cope** with their immediate problems. In addition, they tend to bring a more positive attitude to new situations; in other words, they are **willing** to make adjustments and to **adapt** their perception of stressful situations, in order to decrease their impact.

As an electrologist, I've often treated clients who, in my view, are dealing with stress—at work, in a relationship and with families—yet do not resolve the underlying problems—the circumstances. They keep their resentments bottled up instead. Rather than coping differently with the stress, they internalize the anger and hostility they feel. Their tension is clear, but they are unable to recognize what to do with it, perhaps because they are afraid to deal with it. These clients seem rigidly controlled and are frequently angry or irritable over minor causes. The major source of anger, in turn, remains unexpressed, therefore can't be resolved. In general, when such clients have problems or crises in their lives, they make slower progress with electrolysis and require more treatments.

The client's perception of difficult situations also affects the **progress** he or she achieves with electrolysis. Clients who approach problems **creatively**, with **confidence** in their abilities to find **solutions** and make compromises, will probably grow less hair than those who are closed-minded and unable to adapt. Stress is a part of our daily lives; we all need to learn whatever we can to manage it.

Remember that stress is a human condition, so be **gentle** with yourself. Give yourself time to deal with the current situation; the problem may have taken a long while to develop, so don't expect to **solve** it overnight. The first step is to examine the problem, realistically, and be **aware** that you have the **power** to make changes. Look at the problem itself, not at how awful it is or how it will affect your future. Above all, don't blame yourself because you have problems—a lowered self-esteem will only lead to increased stress.

Instead, ask yourself some questions: Have you dealt with problems like this in the past? If so, what did you do then? Did you **learn** anything at that time that you can apply now?

If the problem is new, what have you used in the past to help you feel **relaxed**, **comfortable** and **confident**? Are there any similarities between the old problem and the new? How have your friends and family dealt with this type of situation? In dealing with new stresses, focus on the specific skills you'll need—be it communication, financial, social or other skills—even stress-management skills. Tell yourself that these **skills** can be learned, and that, with practice, you'll develop them. With time, a new skill will become a habit, and you'll be able to handle current and future problems differently.

Look at the problem from as many angles as you can. And then set priorities. What do you want? What must you do to achieve it? Which aspects of the problem are the most easily solved? Which are the most important? Are you making more difficulties, by comparing yourself with some impossible ideal? Concentrate on actions you can take, and then list the steps to **alleviate** the problem.

Writing out your plan of action gives you a "road map" for handling details and often helps you feel more confident.

The way you think, directly affects your behavior, and though you may not be able to change the world, you can change your attitude toward it. So, tell yourself that you can and will cope. Realize that no difficulty will last forever, and every problem will change with time.

Some people find it helpful just to talk about their tension, whether with friends, family or a therapist. They find, through discussion, that they are able to work through their problems.

Sometimes it helps to get away from the problem for a while. Take **constructive** steps, and use what works for you. Exercise, conversation with friends, walking in the woods, going to the movies, listening to music and taking a vacation are all tried and true ways of getting a break from current pressures. You can also try focusing on some other area of your life for a while, an area where you are **proud** of your **accomplishments**.

The **pampering** you receive in a beauty salon, can also give you a little break, and, feeling happier with your appearance, may give you a psychological **boost**. Or, to help alleviate stress and do something **beneficial** for your body, take yourself to the gym and work out! Get all your toxic thoughts and stress out through your skin pores. Some people feel that sweating does this.

By managing stress in constructive, positive and healthy ways, you'll increase your mental and physical well-being. Discipline yourself. **Retrain** your thought patterns, and decide which emotions you want to feel. As Abraham Lincoln said, "most people are about as happy as they decide to be."

Stress doesn't have to dominate your mind and wreak havoc on your body, *unless you let it*. When minor crises occur, don't just react—*decide* how you're going to react. You can either blow it out of proportion (and increase your stress level), or you can simply deal with the problem as one of life's insignificant, unavoidable mishaps, and move on. Think about it—if you've taught yourself to react to stressful situations in negative, self-destructive ways in the past, then there's no reason why you can't reprogram yourself to react in a positive way now.

Excessive stress is definitely a factor in excessive hair growth and other unwanted health and beauty effects, but sometimes it is far from beyond your control. It is, however, in your power to be happy and control how stress affects you, so don't be afraid to let go of your old thought patterns and make negativity a thing of the past. To quote another great American, Eleanor Roosevelt once said in a famous speech, "No one can make you feel inferior without your consent." The same goes for stress—never forget that **you** are in control of your own mind.

If you are in the middle of conflicts at work, home or anywhere, take the time to resolve matters. If necessary, seek professional counsel. If you keep negative emotions in, your adrenal glands may not be able to handle the results.

Consider These Suggestions

- **Avoid negativity.**

Stay away from people who act, speak and behave negatively, because they can be draining. Find and stick with people who have a positive outlook on life, are **enthusiastic** and **doers**.

- **Breathe deeply.**

Take a couple of minutes, three times a day, to clear your mind and body, by inhaling and exhaling. This will clear your body of stress inducers.

- **Get some sleep.**

The easiest way to stress yourself is to weaken your body's natural defense against it. By exhausting yourself emotionally and physically, you become more open to "The Stress Effect."

- **Stop worrying.**

You can't control everything around you. Be **satisfied** with trying and doing your **best**—nobody can expect more than that. Whatever happens, happens. Live with it; move on and grow **stronger** from it.

- **Stop feeling guilty.**

Many people set up emotional blocks built from guilt and are so busy blaming themselves, they are unable to move forward. You have to find the strength within you to move on—beyond the past you can't change. No good comes from guilt.

- **Relax. Enjoy life, time and scenery.**

Going too fast puts additional stress on your body. This can easily be avoided by slowing down once in a while.

- **Do things the best way you know how.**

Don't stress yourself by trying new methods you aren't comfortable with. Stick to what you know, when you are under deadlines. When you have stress-free time and don't have to worry about the consequences, then you can experiment a little with other things.

POST-WORTHY REMINDERS

"Choose how you want to feel, and focus on something positive to help get you there.
You can redirect your thoughts and not get derailed and depressed by life's stresses and strains."

~•~

"No matter how tough times get, you always have other options and answers."

"A belief is something we give importance to. Keep it in check, when you want to make a change."

~•~

"When you find value in something that is tough or seemingly difficult, you won't find it so hard if you embrace it and grow through it. You learn, earn, and you get beyond it. You can gain lots of benefits from the things you've been through."

~•~

"Be aware: roses are beautiful, but also have thorns. See the truth and take the time to see what you might otherwise miss, before you make a decision too quickly and get pricked. Think about this before you jump into something new."

~•~

"We may not get everything we want, but we won't get anything if we tell ourselves it is impossible.

Be proud of what you have done, instead of thinking that it's never enough.

"Personal hardships and obstacles are merely an opportunity to test your inner strength and wisdom!"

~•~

"We are all capable. Take steps to see your accomplishments."

~•~

PART IV

CIRCUMVENTING THE OBSTACLES

"If you find a path with no obstacles,
it probably doesn't lead anywhere."
— Frank A. Clark

CHAPTER 9

OVERCOMING OBSTACLES TO SUCCESS

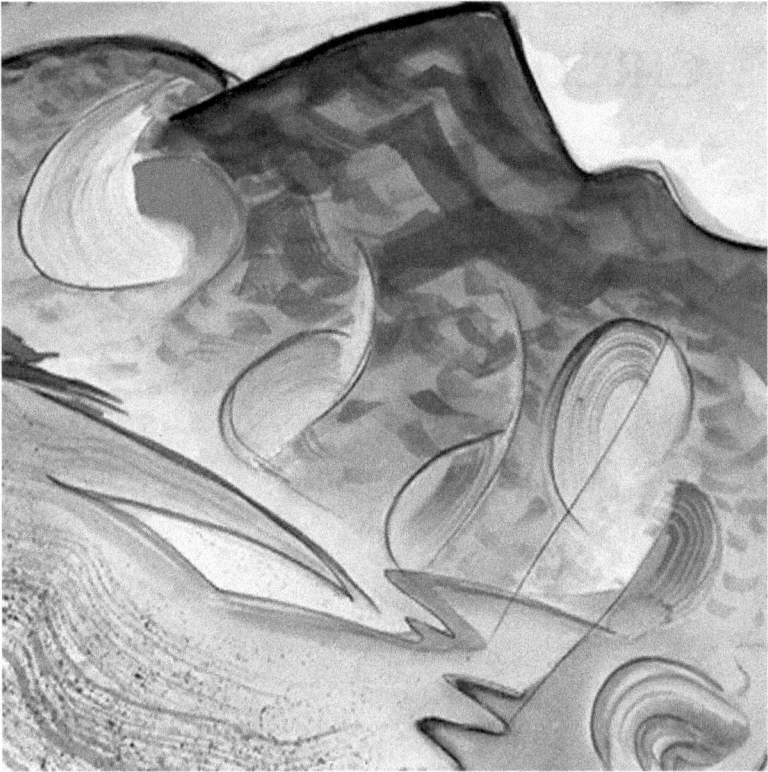

Henry Brown

"Obstacles don't have to stop you. If you run into a wall, don't turn around and give up. Figure out how to climb it, go through it, or work around it."

— Michael Jordan

Negativity can be a way to avoid life's challenges or **advance** toward goal **achievement.** In other words, it can be a form of self-sabotage or a way to deal with our fear of failure. We can choose, instead, to see challenges as **blessings** in disguise. When you face challenges, find a way to **appreciate** them because they will **teach** you a lot.

We can **learn** to view what could manifest as roadblocks, like abuse, stress, fear, daunting tasks and physical challenges, instead, as merely obstacles in the road that we can walk around. We do this by understanding them, confronting them or breaking them down into more **manageable** forms.

EMOTIONAL TRAUMA

ABUSE

As noted earlier, under the summary on "Causes," people don't always decide to be negative. Traumas from the past can leave deep, lasting scars, and negativity is a common result, especially when physical or emotional abuse is involved. Sometimes we must confront the past before we can live in the now and overcome negativity. Not all, but some people who abuse others have been abused themselves. This does not excuse the behavior ; however, it does give us **insight** and **understanding** of the behavior, when we begin to look inward and confront our past trauma. The length of time that people experience abuse, and the type of abuse, can highly impact the way they are affected by it.

Oprah Winfrey's recent report about how past trauma affects thoughts and behavior, is **encouraging**.

Some states are now training healthcare providers, law enforcement officers, and even judges, to understand the importance of asking, "what happened?" to someone who is acting out with bad behavior.

Abuse has many different forms: physical, sexual, emotional, psychological and verbal. Abuse has a wide variety of origins and is not always from parents. And it doesn't just result in abuse of others; it can lead to self-abuse. A common dynamic of an abusive situation involves a power struggle—the desire to have power and control over someone else. This could result from internalization of behavior from previous experience; having a mental illness that involves a feeling of entitlement, meaning a person believes they deserve to have control over another; or even a lack of accountability for actions.

Common mentalities and actions of people who tend to abuse include:

- Thinking you can't be wrong.

- Inability to cope when your feelings are hurt.

- Unleashing emotions physically or by verbally berating someone.

Two more frequent offending tendencies, in relation to abuse, are controlling and manipulating. A very common form of this abusive combination is called gaslighting. This term is used when someone has been psychologically manipulated by another, into believing they are wrong. It comes with the perpetrator's perception that it's ok to subjugate someone else's thinking, into their own—or what they want another person to think.

Another way of putting this would be, telling someone that what they think is true, is *not* true—or making them feel like they are "going crazy." This phenomenon has often been portrayed in the media.

The full effect of gaslighting is created gradually, over time. Sometimes the individual effects are so subtle, they may go unnoticed by the victim, until they begin to believe they are descending into madness.

Have you ever had someone control your life, when you are in a relationship? They may say things like, "You can't see your friends anymore," or they may blame you, accusing you of always misplacing things or saying "you must have forgotten." These are just a few examples. Know that anyone can gaslight; even parents have been guilty of doing this to their children.

I, personally, went through a childhood involving abuse. My father was a very toxic person who exhibited very negative behaviors that he inherited from his family. Unfortunately for us both, he refused to change or even acknowledge his abusive behavior, and he was unable to help me overcome the negative effects that behavior had on me.

Although I hated the things my father did, I was able to see how he was blinded by his negativity.

I had a choice. I could follow in his footsteps, or I could learn to overcome my past and my inheritance. Choosing the latter, I made an active decision to **strive** to become **self-aware** and **mindful** of what I think and say. I took action to prevent myself from repeating the pattern of abuse I had suffered, and you can too. Confronting my past and choosing to identify what my father was doing and understanding why, is one of the best things I've done in my life.

It helped me vet these issues of my father's, before they started to fester and become issues of my own.

If you've ever been on the receiving end of abuse, know you are not alone and, there are those who can help. Read more about ways to help **recover** from trauma, in the section about Post Traumatic Stress.

FEAR

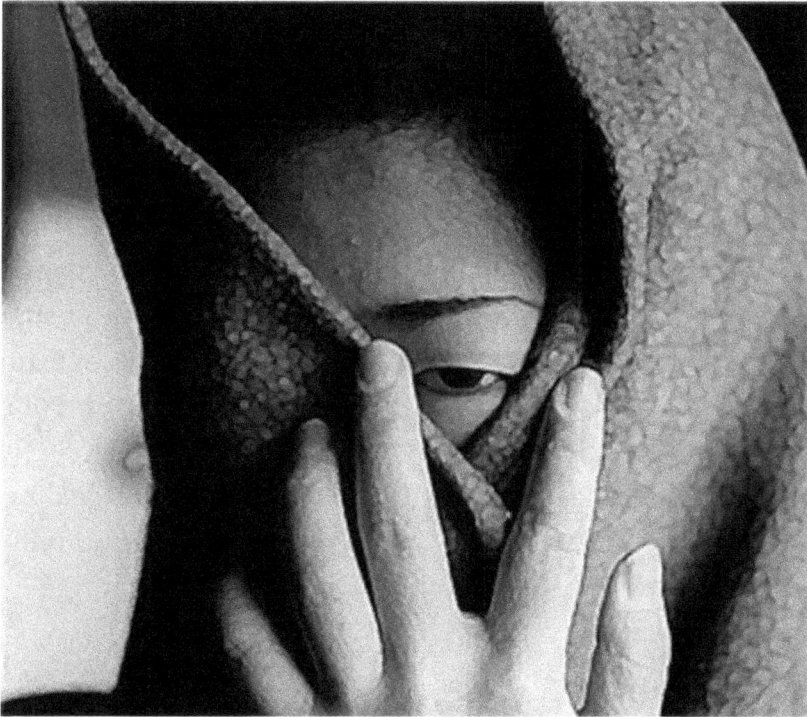

Micah Gampel

"Each time we face our fear, we gain strength, courage, and Confidence in the doing."

—Theodore Roosevelt

Fear, like stress, is a **natural** part of life. It's not a roadblock or a barrier. It's no more than an obstacle that should not stop you from living life fully, just as being shy, should not keep you away from people. You can take **action**, in spite of your fears or other obstacles, simply by moving around them. **Acknowledge** their presence, but keep on walking.

You can eliminate or diminish negative thoughts about yourself, if you learn to confront your fears. This may seem to be a dreary task, but it is necessary for **growth**, and you can learn steps to deal with it.

Though very difficult for some of us, confronting fear does get **easier** after you take the first step, which is simply acknowledging what it is you are afraid of. Then you can use the other tools for overcoming negative thinking, to change the way you perceive, think about and respond to your fears. Use the space at the end of this section to **help** you recognize, the things you fear, by writing them down. Add your thoughts about those fears, if you like.

However, please keep in mind that if you are dealing with past trauma, you may want to put this exercise off until you are more ready to deal with it.

Name Your Fears

This part is up to you. It's just a reminder that sometimes it helps to confront your fears, and to do that, you have to know what they are. This space is for writing them down, when you are ready, and to remind you to do it when you are. It's also for writing your feelings about those fears — and ways you can think of to **overcome** them. But there's no rush. So you decide when it is the right time.

Things I Fear & How They Make Me Feel or Act:

_____

_____

_____

_____

_____

_____

_____

_____

Things I Can Do to Change My Reactions to Fear:

_____

_____

_____

_____

_____

_____

_____

_____

_____

PHYSICAL CONDITIONS THAT CAN CAUSE OR MAKE IT HARDER TO OVERCOME NEGATIVITY

If working to change your thoughts and focus on the positive aspects of a situation seems too difficult or is causing you more stress, you may want to consider getting screened for physical conditions that could impede or challenge your ability to overcome negativity. These include insomnia, nutritional deficiencies, traumatic or other brain injuries, post-traumatic stress disorder (PTSD), physical pain, hormonal and gut imbalances and even exposures to neurotoxins, as in common household products or the outdoor environment. The physical causes can be many, so we will take only a brief look at a few, which are discussed in more detail in this section.

INSOMNIA

Perhaps nothing has more influence on our mood and behavior than our ability to get **sufficient** sleep.

No one who's ever missed a night's sleep—or slept very little for days—can argue the **importance** of **sleep** on your mood, thinking and behavior. As we've already noted, insomnia can be a symptom of many physical conditions, and it can also result from the negativity that increases the stress and anxiety we are dealing with already. When you're ruminating over things that didn't go your way or worrying over things you have to do or things you dislike, your sleep and your overall health can be adversely affected.

So, it's **essential** that we find ways to **relax** and sleep.

And, of course, changing the way we think and the way we focus and face life's challenges will help.

In addition to following the steps to overcome negativity and stress, many found in this book, there are more than a few non-drug options that can be beneficial— nutrients and herbs that can help us relax and improve our ability to fall and stay asleep.

One of these is an amino acid we don't hear that much about and is not as easy to find on store shelves, as most other amino acids. L-theanine is found in green tea and a few over-the-counter supplements. Sometimes combined with melatonin, this amino acid not only helps reduce stress and **enhance** sleep, it is also known to **improve** concentration and even **protect** brain cells against excitotoxicity and electrical activity in the brain associated with anxiety.

According to Jeffrey Castle's report about nutrients that combat stress, results from animal studies show that L-theanine can also help **alleviate** depression. By decreasing anxiety, it can improve concentration and attention.

And there's more. This amino acid is known to reduce the flight-or-fight response, which can raise cortisol (stress hormone) levels, thus improving the heart rate and **protecting** the body from cardiovascular disease. Adding it to caffeine improves cognitive function, with less mental fatigue, while reducing symptoms such as headaches.

As far as dosage goes, you get only about 20 milligrams of L-theanine from a cup of green tea, so you'll probably want to add supplements to get the 100 to 250 daily milligrams needed for anti-anxiety results.

The next effective natural sleep-enhancer that Castle recommends is lemon balm tea, which he says is **prized** by traditional cultures, for its **sedative** effects and its ability to induce sleep. Animal studies with lemon balm extract also found significant reductions in stress and anxiety and improved behaviors of mice that had been conditioned to become fearful. Lemon balm is even used to protect radiology technicians from on-the-job exposures to radiation, and it **boosts** levels of GABA, the relaxation-inducing neurotransmitter. Its components also have the **capability** to protect a person from Alzheimer's disease.

Other **beneficial** herbs used to help with sleep and **relaxation** include Maca and **Holy** Basil. Also, studies using Echinacea Augustifolia, have found this version of echinacea to be as relaxing as a drug sedative, without the unwanted side-effects. Burning two or three bay leaves (done safely in a ceramic dish or metal pan, of course) and allowing this healing smoke to fill a room, is found by some to be very relaxing, even sleep-inducing.

Supplementing with D3, a vitamin in which many of us are deficient, may also be helpful (see more on D3 below). There are other relaxing and sleep-inducing herbs and supplements you may want to look into to see **what works** best for you.

Vitamin D for Insomnia — The Right Kind, The Right Dose

Vitamin D deficiency is linked to many health conditions. One of the latest concerns being discussed, is its connection to insomnia.

Sleep disorders are far from uncommon.

The "Vitamin D Council" estimates that as many as 80 million Americans, alone, struggle with falling or staying asleep, leaving them fatigued throughout most of the day. Prolonged sleep loss can result in more serious health effects, including heart disease and stroke.

The recent research on D is providing hope for insomnia sufferers, because of D's ability to regulate the body's circadian rhythm.

Most or all experts agree that the best source of Vitamin D is the sun. Several say that D2 is *not* the D we need, and it can make insomnia and other conditions worse. What *is* needed is D3. Besides the sun, other natural sources of D3 include wild-caught salmon and mackerel, eggs, cod liver oil and sardines.

Before supplementing with D3, doctors suggest it's best to have your blood levels tested to find the dosage you need to reach optimal levels of 60–80 mg/ml. Dr. Mercola says most of us are likely deficient, and that we should include K2 with any D3 supplement.

Maybe the best part of this news is that we may now have a solution for insomnia and its effects, which eliminates the need for long-term or any use of highly addictive and brain-damaging sedatives or sleeping aids, like the class of drugs known as benzodiazepines and benzo-like drugs. These pharmaceuticals can be far more detrimental to health than disrupted sleep.

PAIN

When we're in pain, especially chronic, severe pain, the last thing we may want to do is work on changing the way we think, even if we know it will help. We may need to deal with the pain and what's causing it, before we can **make headway** in changing any negative thinking tendencies.

Bodily pain may be unrelated to physical actions and, instead, may originate from thought patterns or perception. For example, strained eyes may not be from poor eyesight, but from a dislike of the reading material. Another example: the shock of watching something disturbing on TV, can manifest itself as stomach pain.

As we discussed earlier, pain can be caused by negative thinking, so even when we're in pain, it can't hurt us to try to focus on positive thoughts and **beautiful** or even **funny** things.

Of course, pain is often a symptom of physical problems that warrant medical intervention. If you've already been examined and tested and know the physical cause/s of your pain, but are still experiencing more than is tolerable, you might want to consider the non-psychoactive component of the cannabis plant, known as cannabidiol or CBD, often marketed now in the form of oils, capsules or water-soluble liquids.

Many are reporting that they experience noticeable pain **relief** from using this no-to-very-low-THC version of cannabis. The CBD oil is taken sublingually—a few drops under the tongue, a few times a day. Some NFL players say they use it daily, to get relief from the pain they suffer, from all the hits they experience on the playing field.

CBD oil, often made from industrial hemp, and containing no more than three tenths of a percent of THC, is legal in all U.S. states now and can be ordered online or purchased at some local shops that carry it. An organization called the Realm of Caring (ROC) has information about the latest research on the benefits of using CBD.

Although medical cannabis/marijuana is not legal in some states, even if it contains no psychoactive components (THC), some legal industrial hemp CBD brands have either kept or replaced some or most of the **beneficial** terpenes found in cannabis. If you have questions about which is the **best** hemp or cannabis product to use for pain, you might find very **helpful** a Q&A webinar with Dr. Bonni Goldstein, produced by Manny Goldman, founder of the documentary, "The **Sacred** Plant."

Two studies, one conducted with human subjects at the University of Koln, Germany, and another, using mice at Western University in Toronto, found that CBD increases **anandamides. Ananda** is Sanskrit for **"joy," "bliss"** and **"delight,"** and anandamides, known as the bliss neurotransmitters, are now being investigated for their role in affecting human behavior, including eating and sleeping patterns, and also for pain relief.

Anandamides are already known to inhibit cell proliferation in human breast cancer and for their role in uterus implantation of the human embryo, If you want to learn more about the research on CBD oil and medical marijuana, CNN has produced a very informative documentary available on YouTube, titled "Weed," found here:
https://www.youtube.com/watch?v=Z3IMfIQ_K6U

You can also find out more from The Realm of Caring and about the particular product brands they endorse on their website here: https://www.theroc.us/

BRAIN INJURY—Traumatic or Acquired

Trying to focus on positive thoughts can be very difficult for one who has experienced any kind of brain injury, because repetitive negative thinking, or rumination, is common with brain injury. In fact, suicidal thoughts are said to be six times more common in people who suffered brain injuries.

Rumination can result from the anxiety and depression that is often associated with brain injury, so **alleviating** these, can help break the cycle of negative thinking, which we now know can cause even more brain damage.

Experts say it's best not to just tell someone who suffered a head injury to stop thinking negative thoughts, because doing so can push those negative thoughts to the front of the mind—or to the prefrontal cortex of the brain, to put it more exactly. It has instead been suggested that it's better to help the brain-injured person find an **enjoyable** task that will serve to distract them from negative thoughts. Performing the enjoyable task, will likely, in turn, release **beneficial** chemicals that **promote** more positive thinking.

It will certainly **help** the person **recovering** from brain injury to have positive people around them—those who will remind them of how **strong** and **resilient** they are, to have come through their ordeal—who will treat them like the **heroes** they are.

HORMONAL IMBALANCE

Though not very well known, hormonal imbalances are quite common and occur especially after brain injury. Any kind of jolt to the head can damage the hypothalamus, and this can result in a wide range of changes in personality and the way a person thinks, feels, looks and acts. Like the head injury itself, resulting hormonal imbalances can put up hurdles for a person trying to change negative thinking and even make the person less able to be aware of their own thoughts and actions.

Although believed to be rare, a condition known as hypopituitarism and other pituitary disorders are really not all that uncommon, according to the Pituitary Society. Hypopituitarism is caused by injury to the hypothalamus or pituitary or by radiation, tumors or diseases of the pituitary gland or hypothalamus. The condition is marked by a

117

decreased secretion of pituitary hormones, most of which can wreak havoc on bodily and mental function. Partly due to the eye-opening work by Dr. Mark Gordon, more and more healthcare providers are becoming aware of the need to screen for hormone deficiencies, and places like Gordon's Millennium Wellness Center in Encino, California and Carolina Healthspan in Charlotte, North Carolina are treating these deficiencies with hormone replacement. Carolina Healthspan has also just completed a ground-breaking study, with very **positive** results, using passive neurofeedback to treat NFL players who suffered concussions while playing football.

To simplify, neurofeedback works by increasing the flow of oxygen to the brain, reducing inflammation and **retraining** the brain.

The Hull Institute adds that neurofeedback **heals** and **stabilizes** the brain, making it more susceptible to psychotherapy, which can help heal the mind.

Another method of retraining the brain can be **accomplished** through BrainHQ exercises, anyone with the internet **can** subscribe to and do daily, online. The "brain behind BrainHQ" and the author of *Soft-Wired: How the New Science of Brain Plasticity Can Change Your Life,* is Dr. Michael Merzenich, a **pioneer** in brain **plasticity** research. The yearly subscription to these brain-retraining exercises is very affordable, and you can also try some of the exercises for free here: https://www.brainhq.com

Neurofeedback is one of several non-drug treatments now being used to not only heal or **ameliorate** the effects of brain injuries, but it is also alleviating anxiety, insomnia, depression and other brain-related symptoms, including damage caused by medications and other drugs. Some injured NFL players and parents of autistic children and others with cognitive impairment have also found hyperbaric oxygen therapy very helpful in healing the brain and improving cognitive ability.

We are now learning, through studies done with veterans and from some neuroscientists, that brain injury can result from emotional, as well as physical, trauma. Neurofeedback can help, whatever the cause of the injury.

NUTRITIONAL DEFICIENCIES AND HEAVY METALS

Screening for nutritional deficiencies is another **important** step to consider, if you find you're having trouble focusing on positive thoughts.

Nutritional deficiencies can cause insomnia, anxiety, weakness, lack of energy, and of course they can contribute to negative thinking, which just makes other things worse, as we have learned.

Two very good sources I've found for helping you decide which deficiencies you might want to screen for first, are the United Kingdom's Brain Bio Centre and Dr. William Walsh's website, found here: http://www.walshinstitute.org/

The Brain Bio center's website is found at this url: http://www.foodforthebrain.org/ and has information on how nutrition can improve distressing conditions, like stress, depression, insomnia and even autism or schizophrenia. Dr. Walsh's Research Institute offers information on nutritional needs, to help the mind and body **function optimally,** and offers test kits your doctor can order for you to complete and return for evaluation.

What about heavy metals affecting the way you think? Of course we have all heard by now, due to the Flint, Michigan tragedy, about the adverse effects of lead on the brain. Lead and mercury can have devastating effects on the way the brain develops and functions and, in turn, the way you think and feel. But the **good news** is that there are treatments that help remove heavy metals from the body and even natural ways of **detoxing** them.

Places that offer kits your doctor can order for lead and mercury screening are Genova Diagnostics in Asheville, North Carolina and The Great Plains Laboratory in Lenexa, Kansas.

These labs facilitate testing for healthcare providers who believe in the importance of challenge tests, which they say measure not only recent exposures, but the amount of stored lead, mercury or other metals in the body.

"SWEET MISERY"

Most of us are aware of the **importance** of a good diet and how that affects the way we feel and think—and of course there are the added **benefits** of exercise. But people may not realize how good they would feel, if they simply cut out processed sugar. Aside from managing stress, ditching sugar is the best way to reduce inflammation in the body that can lead to all forms disease and have a negative effect on the brain, says Mark Hymen, M.D. He adds that processed sugar is the "root cause of our obesity epidemic and most of the chronic disease, sucking the life out of our citizens and our economy."

Hymen advises that if we can't or won't drop sugar altogether, we should at least reduce it and not consume it daily. Also, we must give up the worst form of sugar, which is high fructose corn syrup. If you're hooked on sodas and/or consume a lot of high fructose corn syrup, you can begin improving the way you feel and think, simply by giving up this very destructive form of sugar and limiting the more natural kinds. Take time to check the ingredient labels on the sweets you buy, and when you have a craving for something sweet, choose those without corn syrup and with the lowest sugar content.

However, this definitely does not mean you should replace processed sugars with artificial ones. Aspartame, the main Ingredient in several sugar substitutes and in almost all chewing gums found on store shelves, can be very damaging to the brain. Also, very informative, is the documentary film, "Sweet Misery," if you want to know more about the adverse effects of aspartame.

Splenda, even though made from sugar, is chlorinated sugar, and many bad health effects have been reported from people simply working in the factories that produce it. It's important to know that if you decide to give up added sugar completely, and do it cold turkey (abruptly), you will likely experience symptoms of withdrawal the first few days— including irritability and headaches. However, within a week or two you'll likely find the taste of sweets even offensive, and within a month, you may experience a sense of well-being and positivity you never knew existed before.

Try it, or at least learn to sweeten foods with more **beneficial** sweeteners like stevia, maple syrup, xylitol (from birch, not corn) or sorbitol. Maple syrup has the added benefit of at least a little natural iron. Xylitol has the added benefit of **protecting** teeth from decay.

THE GUT-BRAIN CONNECTION AND PROBIOTICS

Recent research is backing up what a number of mostly functional doctors have believed for some time—that there is a gut-brain connection, and unbalanced bacteria in the gut can cause negative thinking, as well as other unwanted symptoms.

One study in the Netherlands, though small, found a significant decrease in negative thought among study participants taking probiotics for four weeks. According to a report on the study by GreenMedinfo, "The probiotic species used in the formula were: Lactobacillus acidophilus, Bifidobacterium bifidum, Bifidobacterium lactis, Lactobacillus brevis, Lactobacillus casei, Lactococcus lactis and Lactobacillus salivarius." Most or all of these are found in yogurts sold in grocery stores.

Yogurt has long been promoted as being good for our digestive health, because it contains probiotics—or friendly bacteria. Yogurt became even more popular, after UCLA researchers, in 2013, found evidence that probiotics, ingested in food, can have a positive effect on human brain function and can even reduce stress.

In other words, it's "a two-way street," says the UCLA Newsroom report on this study. The stress that can lead to digestive problems may actually be alleviated, and other brain symptoms improved, through balancing the bacteria in the gut.

What we don't know from the UCLA study, however, is the quality of the yogurt that was used or which strains or cultures of probiotics it contained. We don't know if this studied version of yogurt contains the same strains of probiotics we would find on the market.

Fact is, not all yogurts are made the same, and regular use of those that are high in sugars or contain artificial sweeteners, GMOs, bovine growth hormones and/or artificial preservatives, can cause more health problems than they alleviate.

What we really want are live probiotics, and yogurt isn't the only natural or always the best source. Probiotics are also gained by consuming kefir, sauerkraut, kimchi, natto, tempeh, raw goat cheese, apple cider vinegar and sour pickles (organic ones). Dr. Axe recommends yogurt as a good source of probiotics, IF it is not pasteurized and "first, that it comes from goat's or sheep's milk, second, that it is grass-fed and third, that it is organic."

While organic yogurt, containing live cultures, and naturally sweetened with added fruits or stevia can be beneficial to healthy people, by keeping their gut bacteria in balance, supplemental probiotics may be needed when candida or other more severe imbalances occur—or when taking antibiotics.

Most yogurt contains Lactobacillus bulgaricus and Streptococcus thermopiles. A few may also include Lactobacillus casei, Lactobacillus acidophilus and Bifidus. However, if we are looking to alleviate depression or stress, for example, two other strains of probiotics, not usually found in yogurt, B. infantis and B. longum, may be what we really need.

Treating cognitive function and conditions like stress and depression with probiotics, is a rather new concept, so you may need to spend some time researching and speaking with nutrition experts, to find a yogurt or supplement that is most beneficial to your health needs.

For more about the study on Probiotics and negative thinking, visit GreenMedinfo's webpage: http://www.greenmedinfo.com/blog/probiotics-reducenegative-thinking

A PHYSICALLY TOXIC ENVIRONMENT—BAD AIR QUALITY

We've all heard about "toxic relationships." But there is another toxic relationship we can have with our environments, the most important being the places where we live and sleep—where most of us spend most of the hours of our day.

With the use of volatile pesticides, perfumes, fabric softeners and candles, many of us are unknowingly poisoning ourselves, little by little, sometimes so slowly we don't even realize it's happening.

One serious concern about this slow poisoning is its effect on our brains. Most of us know that heavy metal poisoning, like lead and mercury exposure at an early age, can do anything from causing developmental disabilities to learning disabilities—creating, sometimes, even a criminal mind. But most of the poisons in our environment are far more subtle than these. However, the good news is that we have **safe alternatives** for all of them. Even better, these alternatives are often more **effective** than their poisonous counterparts.

When we use products that slowly poison our bodies and our brains, we can have trouble thinking and sleeping, and we can also have a harder time dealing with daily or much more severe stress. It can affect our sleep and our ability to relax, as well as weaken our immune system and make us vulnerable to disease and also, in turn, affect our outward appearance.

This information is lately becoming more and more publicized, and therefore we now have access to **affordable,** safer and many **fragrance-free** products. It's no longer necessary to spend a lot of money on these **nontoxic alternatives**, and just knowing which non-toxic older ones to use, can save us even more.

For example, nothing beats white vinegar for cleaning and disinfecting. To disinfect, all you have to do is add hydrogen peroxide to the mix, which is even more powerful when you use vinegar and peroxide separately, spraying one after the other. Free-and-clear laundry products are **essential** to good health, because the others contain highly toxic synthetic fragrances that wear on your sinuses, your brains and your skin. Sleeping on sheets washed in scented detergents and fabric softeners—and dried with scented dryer sheets—is a nightmare for people with chemical sensitivities. Also, these products have been suspected of causing sudden infant death, which may be the reason putting children to sleep on their backs has helped,

There is also research that supports the suspicion that toxic ingredients in dryer sheets, alone, are contributing to or causing bone loss. And the exhaust from dryers, using these toxic sheets, is polluting the outdoor environment, while the clothes contaminated with dryer sheet toxins are polluting the lungs, brains and sinuses of those who wear them— children being the most vulnerable.

My friend's mother planted azaleas near her dryer's exhaust vent, and those plants soon turned brown and died. So, imagine what those fumes are doing to your body—and your brain.

Pesticides are a very complicated issue, but the most important thing to know about them is that most are incredibly toxic, often because of so-called inert, but not listed, ingredients. Taking into consideration what else you are exposed to when you encounter a pesticide, the combination could have a devastating effect on your health, depending upon your individual ability to metabolize and the synergistic effects of combined toxic exposures. For example, a man who'd taken a normal dose of Tylenol died soon after, while he was playing golf on a course recently treated with a pesticide. The Tylenol, still in his system, prevented his liver from protecting him from the toxic pesticide exposure.

Without going into too much more detail, it's important to know that a spray pesticide is far more likely to harm you than a solid or powder (so long as you don't breathe the dust of the powder or eat it).

Boric acid—finely applied, without clumping, or mixed with flour in a shallow pan or other open container— can be more **effective** than any spray pesticide and far less likely to poison you. Ant bait composed of syrup and boric acid (Terro Ant Bait, for example) will stop ants from coming back inside your home, without poisoning you and your family in the process. Just a spray bottle of basic, fragrance-free liquid soap, mixed half and half with water, will kill most bugs on contact, because the soap breaks down their exoskeletons.

For more about how everyday products are poisoning our lives, a recommended film is Jon Whelan's, *Stink*, which grew out of his desire to protect his children from the breast cancer that killed their mother.

For more about the least toxic ways to clean and control pests, you can go to www.pesticide.org and other similar websites that share information on toxic pesticides and their alternatives.

For tips on natural and non-toxic cleaning, you might want to check out Debra Dadd's website and/or books, one titled, "Nontoxic and Natural."

So, if we want to change our negative thinking to positive, it helps to start off with a "thinking machine"—a brain—that's not bogged down or injured with toxins. To help think, feel and look better—to improve your overall quality of life—get these unnecessary toxins out of your environment—permanently!

POST TRAUMATIC STRESS DISORDER

Delayed Emotions after Stressful or Tragic Circumstances

Traumatic events can leave you in a crisis. After a tragic loss, you may not be capable of coping or feeling emotion. This can last for years at a time and can give way to post-traumatic stress syndrome, or disorder, at any moment. It can happen from anything that has affected you deeply, especially something you didn't expect or that really shocked you.

Post-traumatic stress disorder is debilitating and can include symptoms, such as flashbacks of the trauma, depression, insomnia and anxiety—and even suicide. It can lead to negative thoughts and behaviors, including addictive behaviors, like binging and abusing alcohol and drugs. These addictive behaviors are mechanisms we may use to numb feelings or pain or to fill a void—also as defense mechanisms to protect ourselves from the trauma.

Not just a term for emotional symptoms, PTSD is now known to cause physical changes to the brain. It can cause abnormalities in the amount of gray matter versus white matter, upsetting the balance between the two and affecting the way information is processed. This disruption can adversely affect your mood and your memories associated with the past.

In line with negativity, PTSD can lead to blaming innocent parties and displacing or projecting our anger onto others.

How can you stop this before it starts? Seek out a well-recommended therapist who understands trauma, as soon after the tragic event as possible, to help you deal with what happened. Keeping a journal to express your feelings, may help you get through the mourning process. However, as Dr. Bessel van der Kolk suggests, it may be best to find a physical way to calm down your stressful feelings, *before* you can deal with confronting the trauma. Know that even if a traumatic experience is not affecting you immediately after it happens, its effects still might appear later in life.

If PTSD does appear, there are now new **therapies** being used, which specifically target PTSD. They include neurofeedback, eye movement treatments, known as EMDR and Brainspotting, specially designed breathing exercises and trauma-sensitive yoga, to name a few.

Dr. van der Kolk helps people suffering from PTSD at The Trauma Center in Boston, and he has written a book, *Traumatic Stress: The Effects of Overwhelming Experience on Mind, Body, and Society*, about how to deal with the effects of trauma.

In a more recent book, *The Body Keeps the Score: Brain, Mind, and Body in the Treatment of Trauma*, he explains how traumatic stress can literally rewire the brain, especially those
areas that focus on **pleasure**, **trust** and control.

The **good news** is that this damage does not have to be permanent. There are new, **innovative** ways to treat it that don't rely on drugs. These areas can be **healed,** through **treatments** like those mentioned above, which are also beneficial to those suffering concussions and other brain injuries. Van der Kolk also recommends what he calls play and **mindfulness** therapies and other alternatives, as opposed to drugs and talk therapies, which he says are often not useful for those suffering from PTSD.

MORE ON STRESS

Although it may seem repetitious, we just can't say enough about the impact of stress and ways to manage it.

Some doctors are **aware** that unresolved stresses from our past can affect our health in the present. For some, it is an emotional distress, such as anxiety or depression, or a physical effect, such as chronic, defined, or unexplained pain. Whatever the symptom, coming to grips with and releasing an old trauma, often **clears up** health problems and unexplained pain.

One **enlightened** doctor suggests that both humans and animals have built-in mechanisms that allow them to bounce back, to cure themselves from old wounds. He believes in using positive **stimulation,** through physical movement, mental exertion and emotional activity to help allow the mind and body to **recover**.

It is important that you are **comfortable** with yourself in the present. If some part of your past is unresolved, talking to someone may help give you **closure**. However, be aware that just dumping your thoughts on others, puts more stress on both of you. If even telling the story can produce these negative and upsetting feelings, you might be better off trying to vent with someone who can actively listen and help intervene and provide support.

Focus on **self-forgiveness**. If you are taking anger out on yourself, because you believe you have mishandled something, it's time to **forgive,** with self-healing messages. Try finding ways to comfort yourself, before seeking outside stimulation to **cure** the problem. Be the solution. If something upsetting happens, it doesn't have to rule your life. You have a **choice** to change now or at any other given moment.

During difficult times we don't have to feel bad about having problems. Instead of "living inside" an issue, work around it, and turn dark moods or thoughts around.

POINTS FOR POSITIVE CHANGE

Unnerving as it is, stress can also **motivate** us to be productive. It's important to remind ourselves that:

- **Individuals can be ingenious and very creative**.
With all this **intelligence**, why do we sometimes put walls in our way? There's no reason to let a problem cut us off or slow us down. There is always a way to get through or around any obstacle or to overcome any situation. We just have to think about what we can do to get started.

- **We can learn by doing.**

Try using the **energy** of stress, **productively,** to your advantage. Find something of **value** from a crisis. Don't let stress effect your internal and external life, making you unprepared for challenges. Instead of letting it debilitate your physical and emotional body, take the energy that goes into stress, and **harness** and **redirect** it to help you, instead of hold you back.

• **Through management and controlling the effects of stress, we can learn to get through it all.**

Go from victim to **victorious,** by **discovering** your unknown **power.**

REDIRECT STRESS AND ANGER TO POSITIVE ACTIVITIES

Find an activity you like, and motivation will follow.

Positive self-expression is healthy. Many individuals who didn't have supportive parents as role-models, have expressed themselves through art, which sometimes shows their belief system in how they treat themselves

With Van Gogh, everything was heavy, textured and layered. Renoir's imagery was romantic. Then there are artists who twist themselves inside out, to come up with their own personality, like Chagall and Picasso. Salvador Dali was thoroughly driven—can you imagine being in a relationship with him?

You can often tell by the colors people use, by the jewelry they wear and/or by the way they carry themselves,

132

whether or not they're **self-nurturing, independent** and/or **confident** in their opinions and views of the world.

- **Set Achievable Goals.**

You don't have to tackle a problem all at once. By breaking down a difficult task into smaller portions, you can manage something immense, step by step. **Self-motivation** reaps **rewards**. The merit you give yourself for even a small job, well done, can **propel** you further toward overall success.

- **Have a Supportive Belief System.**

Choose one that works for you, not against you. If the one you have doesn't work for you, find one that does. Although it doesn't necessarily happen as quickly as you'd prefer, changing your beliefs is possible. Don't put a time limit on what you need to change.

Change happens when it happens. When you don't put pressure on yourself, it's bound to happen more easily.

- **Learn to Relax.**

Doing so, may not always make change happen faster, but, more than likely, it will. It helps me to repeat a mantra to myself such as, "It will get done."

- **Redirect Anger.**

Try to discover the unconscious patterns in yourself, and find more effective responses to them. One of the most damaging of these is anger.

Anger can be tricky. It harms us and others, if we suppress it, and it does the same. if we hold on to it or express it inappropriately.

Many women tend to get "prune lips" or lip lines, from withheld or unreleased anger or thoughts. Not only do our facial muscles constrict, but our body experiences this same side effect.

We've all heard of jaw clenching, which is most often produced from stress and, invariably, a negative perception and suppressed anger. My article called, "Double exposure: Stress in Your Mind and in Your Skin," goes more deeply into this topic.

Did you know you punish yourself and others, when you hold on to a grudge or anger for a long time? You may not realize the amount of time you lose that could have been utilized on more pleasurable opportunities. The more time you spend talking about an upsetting situation or point of view, the more its power can escalate within you. There are many reasons why learning how to let go of anger is very valuable. Prolonged anger gets in the way of **effectiveness** and causes toxicity in our bodies, from which we will need to **recover**. Frequently, anger wreaks havoc on your body — causing diarrhea, headaches and other ailments, even depression. This self-imposed stress does not serve you.

Anger also interferes with **communication**. But when we step back and learn to approach another without blame, they will more likely hear us. Otherwise, they become focused on our tone and body language, picking up on the negatives, instead of what's being said. This causes further detachment and indifference. Reaction to our anger is more likely to result in escalating, rather than solving the problem.

You don't want to give others a reason to avoid your company. Learn how to consciously redirect your thinking, and choose to limit the duration or intensity of your anger. When you have every reason to get angry, don't. Make a conscious decision not to.

We don't have to forgive someone to approach them without hostility, even though it can be hard to approach someone **lovingly,** if we feel hurt or mistreated by them. Oftentimes, we become attached to our anger, and we let it grow into something larger. Rather than moving on from it, we dwell on it, and it festers, becoming an even bigger issue than it was to begin with. Rather than holding on to negative thoughts and feelings, learn when to brush them off and focus on more important things. Anger's energy can be used positively to get things done, instead of turning inward, causing physical distress, or outward, on others

The key is to acknowledge the anger, and then redirect it, so that it doesn't become a further catalyst for negativity and harm. Also "anger" evolves from a negative perception, therefore one can clean up the negative thoughts, before they escalate into anger.

- **Let Go of Emotional Pain.**

Minimize pain, by **relaxing** and letting go of your attachment to it. The past is unchangeable; our only real option is to move forward and detach from the pain. This permits a **clearer** mind. Don't hurt yourself with self-defeatist thoughts.

When someone hurts or disappoints you, thank them—or at least be **thankful**—for their giving you opportunity to develop overcoming resources within yourself. You may not be happy about this idea, but a little pain teaches us to deal better with other wounds. By thanking them, you won't hold onto the anger; you will instead minimize it and redirect your attention to places that **benefit** you better.

THOUGHT MANAGEMENT

Perception has a great impact on how you deal with stress. Imagine you're late and stuck in traffic. One reaction would be to curse your luck and to generate stress about something that you are unable to change.

However, did you ever think you could also perceive the same event as private time, to reflect or **relax**? Point: go with the flow.

We all need help figuring out how to get through loss, death, breakups and toxic attachments. Chaos presents new difficulties. It's up to us to decide the amount of time we want to spend feeling bad. It isn't a waste, but rather a **learning experience**. By thinking about situations in a more positive light, we can begin reorganizing our lives and get through the crises.

WORD CHOICES AND RELANGUAGING

The words we use are very important. Words have **power** to raise our self-esteem and to drop a lot of heavy, negative, emotional baggage. However, when you use words like "forever" or "never," you close off possibilities. I used to get very upset when I couldn't finish something and felt as if there would never be a resolution. A few simple words changed this negative thinking. Instead of saying "I can't finish this," I say, "I can't finish this *yet* or now." It was an accident, but it set me **free**.

Speaking once on The Oprah Show, sharing her **revelations** about the use of words, Iyanla Vanzant told her audience that "Words create experiences. Words are things, So, when you say I can't, you won't." This reminds me of what a friend's mother used to say, many times, "Can't never *could* do anything."

Paula Potts, who wrote. *Yesterday When I Was Crazy: A Sacred Contract with Healing*, says she benefited tremendously from Ivanla's and her own mother's advice, She advises us to "Give this idea of relanguaging some thought" and see the "difference you feel when you **soften** your expressions about your life experiences. She reminds us to be **"gentle"** with ourselves in the process, using **"healing words and loving thoughts."**

Practicing relanguaging techniques, before going to sleep, can be very helpful. Planting **pleasant** dreams for yourself can help you wake up **happier and healthier**. Consider suggestions like: "Somehow things are going to work out," "It's not the end of the world," "I'll be able to find a way," "There are a lot of things going great in my life," "This will work out in time" and "I don't have to be thinking about bad things now; I'll take care of it tomorrow."

CONSIDER THE "YET" FACTOR

Fear and worry can be extinguished by taking advantage of the "yet factor." For example, the thought, "I will never meet him," seems painfully certain. Consider rephrasing that thought to "I haven't met him *yet*." Doing so alleviates hopelessness. You may not have finished your work, causing you anxiety, but realizing you haven't finished it *yet*, decreases tensions.

Another way to explain this is: when I say, "I don't know," it feels like there's nothing more I am able to find out, or that I am shutting myself down to other answers and possibilities. Instead of limiting yourself in this way, take a minute to think about what you feel that you don't know. Then realize that you can change or avoid needless suffering, by simply adding one word, "yet."

Changing the words or thoughts to "I don't know **yet,**" lets you relax a little. With the belief that you will *find* other possibilities, options, etc., you *will* find the answers you're looking for.

It's amazing how you can stop the recurring mind chatter and self-defeating anxiety, by making this one simple adjustment in your thought process. Delays and challenges are part of life. We have to learn that there is a way out, around or through most obstacles. I have side-stepped many problems, just by knowing that I can shift my belief system,

To turn things around and give yourself a sense of peace and a level of certainty, add the word "**yet.**"

TRANSFORM PAINFUL MEMORIES

With practice, you can transform painful memories into **powerful** resources that you can use for the present and the future.

Focusing attention on the past, is not going to help you move forward into the future. It's times like those that you think it could have been done differently, but nothing you do is going to make a difference, other than seeing the growth from the past and your situations. It's good to realize that part of you needed to be healed. Then you need to acknowledge whether or not that experience made you get stronger.

By looking back, can you see how many miles you've come. Start with the present. If it is colored by a troubled past, making it more acceptable to you will help you **believe** in and experience **a better** future. Realize that NOW is all you really have. You can choose now to be the master of your own mind, take charge of your reactions, or take no action and risk getting the same results as before.

Know that at any given moment, you have the opportunity to relieve or lesson the negative impact of an event on your body and your mind and focus on something worthwhile. If things improve now, they can continue to get better tomorrow. It's important to realize that our past is not necessarily a reflection of who we are. Our experiences, even the hard ones, are **valuable,** in that they help teach us not to repeat mistakes. Even when we do, we must put those mistakes in the past and get back on the path to present and future.

Just having the will to improve, can help you begin to free yourself from the burdens of the past. No one can change what has already happened, but you can change your perception of an event and **dare** to **improve** the road for the future.

HOW TO GET THROUGH IT ALL

Everyone has the resources for whatever they really want, but they have to find the **motivation** within, to access them. **Support** groups help us grow self-esteem and a broader perception. Get motivated, and find supporters! The additional support **bolsters** a stronger sense of **confidence,** which provides extra **energy** and **strength** to help you grow. Your **spiritual** side might **enjoy tai chi,** short for t'ai chi chuan. It is the gentlest of the martial arts, often called "meditation in motion." You can **strengthen** your mind and body, by exercising your inner energy, or "chi." This practice improves muscle strength, **flexibility** and **balance**, which helps combat insomnia and stress. The benefits are experienced as both an emotional **release** and a sense of inner strength.

Examined objectively, stress can be seen as just one of several obstacles we encounter in life. You can minimize or eliminate stress, by using techniques to calm you down or manage stress, by breaking down large tasks into smaller components. The power to turn negatives into positives is within us all, and the **ability** to confront your problems is very strong. Minimizing and managing stress, will make it **easier** to take charge and change your future!

PART V

RELATIONSHIPS

"We've got this gift of love, but love is like a precious plant. You can't just accept it and leave it in the cupboard or just think it's going to get on by itself. You've got to keep watering it. You've got to really look after it and nurture it." — John Lennon

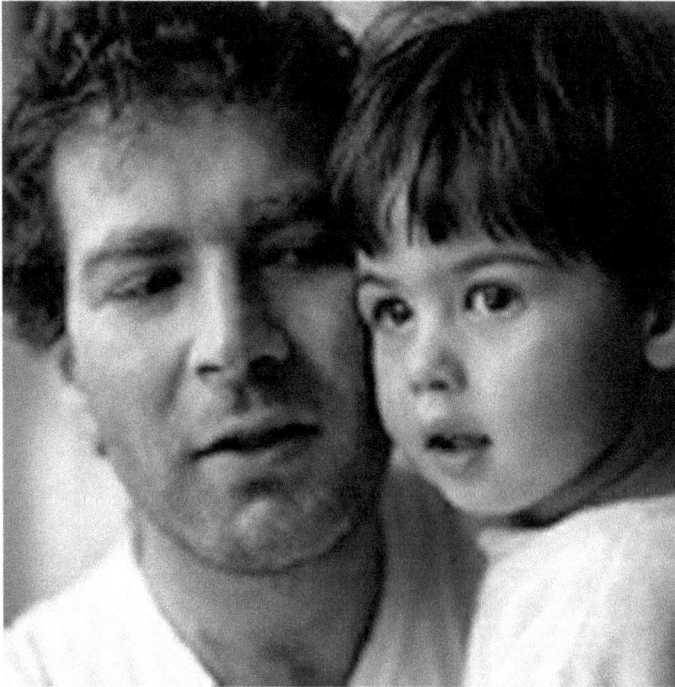

Micah Gampel

142

CHAPTER 10

IMPROVING RELATIONSHIPS BY
OVERCOMING NEGATIVITY

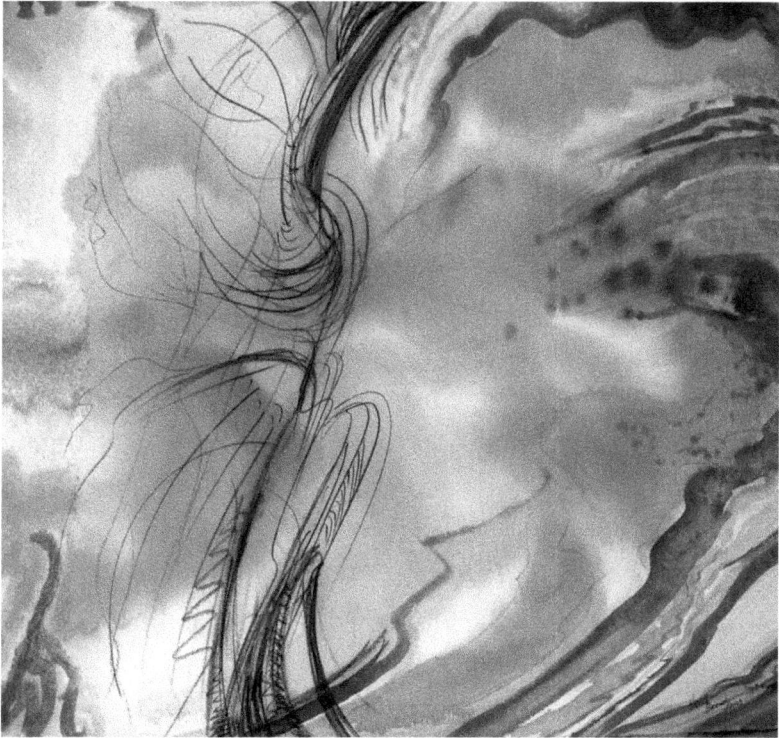

Henry Brown

"How people treat you is their karma; how you react is yours."
— Wayne Dyer

So far, we've discussed mainly how changing your perspective and the way you think, can improve the way you feel and your **happiness** and **self-esteem.** Now we will further **explore** how those changes can help improve your actions, as how they relate to personal and professional relationships.

CURING OUR OWN TOXICITY

Though it may be hard to realize or admit, you can be the main contributing factor to the toxic behaviors in your relationships.

Dr. Daniel Amen has coined the phrase, "Automated Negative Thought" or ANT. ANTs, in turn, produce negative behavior. However, when we identify this, we can unlearn the pattern. Some examples of ANTs are those discussed earlier. They are: thinking with our feelings, always-or-never feelings, fortune telling, mind reading and blame. These are all fairly common ANTs that many people experience and oftentimes struggle to overcome. Sometimes we learn about our negativity, by examining the way our friends and partners react to us, which can be one of the best indicators that we need to change.

Both **romantic** and platonic relationships go through periods of negativity. Sometimes these can deteriorate into toxic relationships. However, identifying the sources of negative thinking, including our own contribution, is an important factor in **improving** our relationships.

This section predominantly focuses on romantic relationships; however, much can be applied to relationships that are just platonic or familial.

Consider communication. Have any of your partners ever found it difficult to open up to you?

Maybe they were worried about your reaction or whether or not you would present yourself to them in an accessible way. When we communicate with others, we need to try to be **open-minded** and **reflective** of the situation. It's not always about doing the right or wrong thing; it's about being able to be **flexible** in the situation and to react proactively, instead of giving a stagnant response.

If you are always expecting the other person in the relationship to bring up issues or begin a discussion, you are not actively participating with them. You are simply not making the effort needed to maintain the **balance**.

In times of vast change in our relationships, it can be difficult to effectively communicate with our partner. When we emotionally distance ourselves from our partners, we end up building a wall surrounding us. This blocks our communication and hinders any progress. However, by establishing and continuing an **open, receptive, two-way** communication between you and them, it can help guide you through whatever obstacle or issue your relationship is facing.

Remember that blaming someone else, and especially insulting them, doesn't solve anything—it's one of the most obvious signs that you are in a negative mindset. And sometimes the root of the problems in the relationship is our own doing. Learn how to express your thoughts and concerns, without transferring blame to your partner. Voicing our thoughts and feelings, **effectively** and **mindfully,** is an important step we can take to help overcome these challenges. Being **productive** in your communication style, without blaming another, is more **solution-oriented**.

It's important that you try to **resolve** issues, rather than being critical. Be open to feedback. Be **true** to yourself; always own your own feelings, instead of assuming someone else's. When you want to help someone else, know that you have to fix your own negative issues first. If you can't **solve** your own problems, how can you **hope** to help someone else solve theirs?

Nevertheless, know that you are **worth giving** and **receiving love** and **companionship**. You've heard it said, "We get the love we think we **deserve**." You might want to look into understanding yourself first. However, know you are **capable** of a healthy relationship.

I'm sure you've heard the following suggestion many times, but most of us find ourselves forgetting how important it is. Learn to use "I" instead of "YOU" statements, when communicating. Instead of making a blaming statement like, "You always forget to put your clothes away," try saying, "I feel better when the room is not so cluttered. **Please** put your clothes away."

By using "I" statements, and clearly asking for what you need, you take the blame off of someone else and take responsibility for your own emotions. It is an important tool to use to communicate with your partner and anyone else. It introduces **discussion** and opens up **dialogue,** instead of shutting things down. You become much more **clear** when talking about your emotions and feelings, when you use "I" statements.

ACTIVE LISTENING

Another crucial part of effective communication is active **listening**. This involves actually trying to comprehend what someone else is saying, as opposed to just letting it go in one ear and out the other. Many times, we overlook the little things that can give us **the key to understanding** the real issue.

Make sure to comprehend, retain and respond to what is being said, rather than what you want or decide to hear. Often people will take what is said and make it about themselves, instead of who it may have been about, spinning it into their own issue and problem.

In his recent article about the "5 reasons relationships fail," Bryan E. Robinson, PhD discusses what he calls "terminal relationship gridlock." This "gridlock," he says, comes from one or both partners getting stuck in their own point of view, unwilling to consider the other's perspective. This kind of attitude usually results in communication that is not only one-sided, but also "presumptive, heavy-handed and parental" in nature. It comes from a "complete disregard for what our partners might think or feel about important relationship issues, and it can lead to the kind of abusive language and behavior that can be fatal to relationships.

Robinson goes on to elaborate on the kinds of toxic behavior and communication that can end up as "terminal relationship gridlock."

These are:

- Mind Reading—jumping to conclusions about what our partner is doing or thinking, before getting all the facts.

- Emotion Reading—Concluding how our partner feels about something, without asking.

- Name-calling—using "you" statements, instead of "I" statements.

- Put-downs—Criticizing instead of using "I" statements.

- Commanding—Telling a mate what to do, as if you're the boss, instead of a partner.

Constant criticism of a partner almost inevitably results in defensiveness, stone-walling and finally contempt—a recipe for relationship failure.

However, says Robinson, failure is not inevitable if we can remember the simple principles of "consideration, kindness and generosity." These are not only simple and obvious, but they are also backed by science, he adds. Scientific studies, along with Robinson's suggestions for preserving relationships, are completely in line with my own recipe and tips for success, described above. Robinson also recommends "active listening." He explains that "Putting yourself in your partner's shoes, by temporarily suspending your own perspective, sharpens your listening skills and deepens your understanding of their thoughts and feelings, without the need to agree or disagree."

This kind of empathic communication "softens tension" and keeps us from "falling into the trap of who's right and who's wrong," adds Robinson. You can read Robinson's full article on *Psychology Today's* website at the following url: www.psychologytoday.com/us/experts/bryan-erobinson-phd

A BIT MORE ABOUT BLAME

Blame is such a destructive and negative force for both the giver and receiver, that it can destroy relationships, as noted above. For this reason, I will give it a bit more **attention**.

As already noted, the negativity we build inside ourselves can show itself, in the form of blame. Many times people use blame as a coping mechanism, to hide their own feelings of helplessness or vulnerability from someone else. These emotions are very scary and sometimes hard to comprehend. Being able to say, "I am not in control," can be very hard. However, using blame to avoid facing these fears, and what may have caused them, will impair your ability to overcome them and to lead a more **fulfilling** life.

Placing blame is not always a sign of negativity, however. In certain situations, someone *else is* actually at fault. So, it's **okay** to place blame when it's **justified**—if done in a **nonjudgmental** way. However, if you find yourself constantly blaming others for almost everything that happens, this should be a warning sign that there's work for you to do.

Below are some ways I find effective, in helping rid ourselves of toxicity and toxic relationships:

- **Listen** to people when they are trying to tell you something.

- **Strengthen** self-awareness: become aware of the actions we take and how they affect others.

- **Focus** on positive thinking: use tools and suggestions under "Solutions" and from elsewhere, to help change your perspective on situations.

- **Seek** out your own help; be **receptive** to suggestions.

- **Ask** for help from a friend or family member; it's never too late or too early for this; admitting we need help can be scary, but sometimes it's necessary.

- **Consider** professional help; sometimes we need this. It should include screening for physical causes of negative thinking and actions.

- **Limit** time spent with other toxic people; you may need to distance yourself, at least until you have a better grasp on your own toxicity; this can include family members.

- **Find** a motivation partner. Report your action steps to each other. This way you're likely to do more.

One more point I want to make is that we must avoid self-blame, when we realize we are responding in a negative way. Instead of getting down on ourselves, we need to step back and be patient. To do otherwise, will only add more negativity and stress. While we're growing and moving toward change, we can't become an obstacle in our own paths, by being hard on ourselves. We will improve more quickly, if we withhold judgment against ourselves, as well as others.

OVERCOMING NEGATIVITY IN THE WORKPLACE

Negative attitudes can plague workplace productivity. It's proven that emotions can spread from one person to the next, and that negative attitudes lead to less productivity than positive ones. Much like an acid, negative attitudes can melt down others, more easily than positive ones. However, whatever level your position in a workplace, you can turn this around, even when it seems hopeless.

As a supervisor or manager, learn to stay **goal-oriented** when problems arise. Actively **listen** to workers' concerns and problems. Let them vent, to help them **relieve** some of the tension, but don't derail the topic at hand too much.

When approaching someone else about how they might be affecting you and your ability to perform, I find it's a good idea to focus on the positives. People are more **receptive** to receiving positive feedback. Try giving them two **compliments** for every constructive criticism.

Avoid referencing "you," instead of "we" or "us." Using only "you," places blame on one person. If you open yourself up to discussion of an event or situation, you will be much more likely to **resolve** it.

Try to be specific about what it is you want to discuss, instead of being vague. With more **clarification**, those you are trying to reach may be more conscious of the action or thought process behind what you are saying.

Keep in mind that it's human to feel, react and be angry, but your behavior is what's most important. You don't have to take out your feelings on others; find a way to deal with them that is not destructive or hurtful.

PART VI

GETTING TO THE TOP
& STAYING POSITIVE

"For every disciplined effort, there is a
multiple reward
— Jim Rohn

CHAPTER 11

REMINDERS, REWARDS AND RESILIENCE

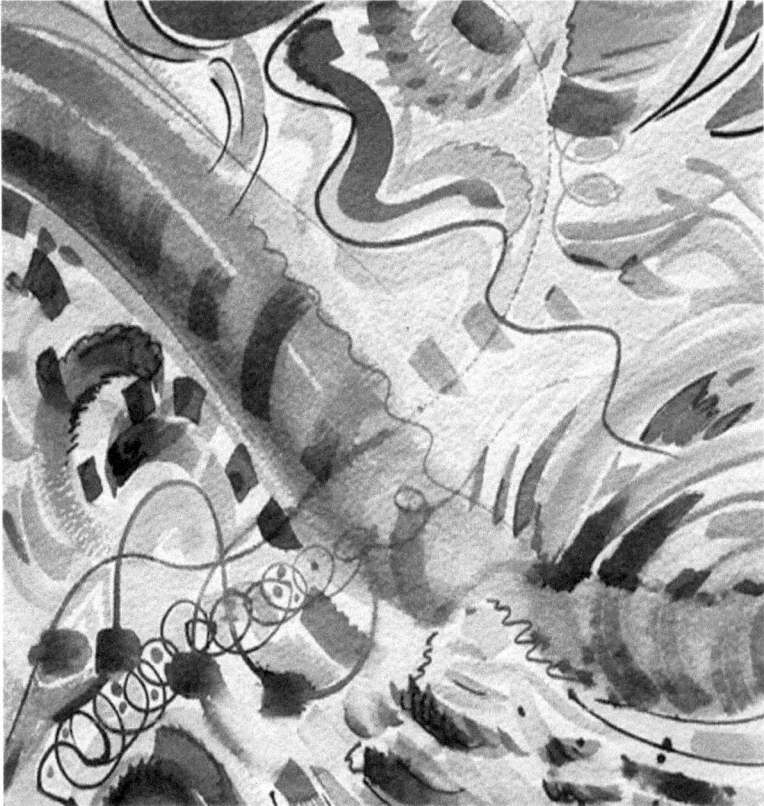

Henry Brown

"Persistence and resilience come from having been given the chance to work through difficult problems."

—Gever Tulley

You've come this far, and that means you've come a long way. You've learned a lot about what causes negativity and how to overcome it, and you've either begun your climb up to "Yes," or you're **willing** to start. **Hopefully** you have taken some steps already. Things are becoming **clearer**, and your thoughts are **calmer**.

Keep in mind that negativity is not an indictment. Although it is part of life, it doesn't have to control your life. If you can recognize it and confront its causes, you can **overcome** it and live a fuller, **happier** existence.

Also remember that no one is keeping time. Work at **improvement** at your own pace. We are all individuals, with different stories and experiences, and some of us have more to overcome than others. It's **okay** to step aside for a while to gather yourself.

Try your best to evaluate your **progress,** without being hard on yourself. You are allowed, even expected and **encouraged,** to give yourself time to grieve and deal with emotional problems.

Time will allow you to deal with these issues more easily, and from there you can move forward to dealing with your negativity. Sometimes you will feel like you're at the bottom, but, like they say, the only way to go, from there, is up. Give yourself this time to express your emotional distress as much as you want. Let it all out; it's okay to cry. Sometimes a punching bag can work wonders.

Try talking to someone you're close to—someone you can **trust** with your feelings. Trying to figure out everything by yourself is hard work; it's never a bad idea to ask for help.

Everyone has the right to vent, but, at some point, you need to **invent**. You need to **develop** ways to better **manage** your stress and negativity. Look for **solutions**.

Consider the tips and information provided in this book. **Learn** from these and my experiences, and **give** yourself the **gift** of a happier, more **fulfilling** life.

Finally, while on your journey to a more positive way of living, remember to be **good** to yourself. Be patient with yourself and treat yourself just as you would someone you greatly **admire** and **appreciate**.

~•~•~•~•~•~•~•~•~•~

POST-WORTHY POINTS TO REMEMBER

~•~

Failure is a **universal experience** that everyone goes through, and accepting this will only make you a **stronger** person.

~•~

Whatever you hold on to, holds on to you. Let go.

~•~

Your mind creates everything you do.

Negative results don't have to be permanent.

~•~

The thoughts and beliefs you choose affect your perception.

~•~

If today is unpleasant, remember tomorrow is another day.

~•~

Thinking and **believing** we can change, opens up **possibility** and **creativity**.

~•~

The road to **happiness** is paved with **strategies** and **solutions**.

~•~

Something **good** comes from everything.

~•~

You can **master** any tough predicament you are in.

~•~

There are 24 hours a day. Every day is a **chance** to grow.

~•~

Sometimes **believing** is **doing**.

~•~

All are born with the same opportunity to make a difference.

TAKE ACTION

- Actively practice and perceive positivity.

- Start being good to yourself, in an organized and **deliberate** way.

- **Permit** yourself to be **adored**.

- **Choose** to learn from an unhappy experience or situation.
- Act instead of react.

- Feed your mind **accurate** and **useable** information.

- Get all the facts before you act or react.

- Challenge yourself.

- If something's not important, let it go.

- Focus on active **recovery**.

- Let deprivation serve you.

- Write down **positive affirmations,** and place them where you can see them every day.

- Use the past to prepare for future events.

- Get over grudges.

- Take notice of what is good, and remember the importance of gratitude.

TAKE RESPONSIBILITY

- Start now; don't wait for tomorrow.

- Commit to daily practice of replacing "no's." with "yeses." But keep it **honest**—say **yes** when you mean yes and no when you mean no.

- When overwhelmed, break projects into **manageable** pieces.

- Give **forgiveness** a chance.

- Look for reasons to be **grateful**.

- Believe you can.

- Give yourself **realistic** goals.

- Pursue **Healthy** Decisions—earn your "PHD."

- Decide you will do what it takes to bring you **closer** to your goal.

- Live in the moment; do your **best** as you see it now.

- Be honest with yourself.

- Go on being **kind**, no matter what happens.

- Never give up.

- Accept that you don't always have to be right.

- Make long-term **success** your goal—not just instant gratification.

After all your efforts to turn negativity into positivity, congratulate yourself. Now you can have more control over your life, because you have chosen to divert your attention from the negative.

~•~•~•~•~•~•~•~•~

REWARDS AND RESILIENCE

Overcoming negative thinking is a **gift** that keeps on **giving,** far more **priceless** than anything any credit card can buy. When we experience the success we get from positive thinking, that generates more positivity and even more success, along with **happiness, peace** and **improvement** in the way we look and feel. It gives us the gift of **resilience.** As we **conquer** our fears, our bad moods, our trauma, our

161

past and our insecurities, by cultivating **positive** thoughts and actions, we develop a **resiliency** to what lies ahead. We are able to face the present and the future, armed with the tools we need to accept or change anything that comes our way, with a **bonus** of feelings of **gratitude** for all the positive and **beautiful** things and aspects of living that we begin to see, maybe for the first time in our lives.

People who are **resilient** have developed an ability to **bounce back** from bad or traumatic experiences and a **flexibility** that helps them **adapt** to present and future stressful situations. They are those who have trained themselves to **overcome** our evolutionary tendency to be negative and who, in turn, are more **optimistic** and **energetic** and **open** to new experiences.

Once you've taken the steps leading to positivity, you may be ready to run the "marathon" of resilience. Running an actual marathon can be a metaphor for resilience, and it can also help to **enhance** or **achieve** this important asset. Studies have shown that traits like hope, self-efficacy, self-understanding and self-control can all be developed and enhanced by running. Runners never know what will come up next in front of them, but the goal is to always **prevail**.

Training yourself to get through the roughest miles and the walls of a marathon, often through trial and error, is much like assessing and doing what you need to do to retain ability to bounce back from the trials and miles of life.

When you're running the marathon to resilience, says Duke clinical social worker Vickie Leff, you want to be **mindful** of your **commitment** and develop **insights** and habits that will take you all the way through the finish line, not just past the first water stop.

When using running, itself, as a stress reliever and tool to resilience, start early; don't wait until the stress is debilitating, before you are motivated. And, as you go the distance, use this opportunity to **reflect** upon how running is helping you deal with other aspects of your life.

When you find challenges, find a way to **appreciate** them, because they will teach you a lot. If you have only a room to live in, you can make it work and find **possibilities** where there seemed to be none, if you can just change the way you think.

I was able to make this work for myself. I have been through the beginnings and the endings of many things in my life; we all have.

This isn't going to be my final chapter. It is my nature to **improve** and **make the most of** what I have been given.

As a student of life, I developed timeless, **enlightening** information to **cushion** our voyage through this earthly existence—sometimes through rough seas, with all its low and high tides. I have chosen to **share** ways I have navigated and **weathered** the storms of life, hoping this will **brighten** the lives of other passengers. My latest storm, the devastating fire in my apartment, did not destroy me, and even spared some of my most **valuable** possessions. It was no accident that I **recovered,** emotionally, from my traumatic childhood and the recent disasters, by helping other people, and I continue to go on doing that. I made my **peace** and created this purpose, so that I didn't feel helpless. I knew I needed to look outside myself, to move away from my own catastrophic circumstances.

And you can too. You *can* modify the way you think and the way you respond. You can start all over again and do things differently. **Believe** you can **overcome** negativity. You have the tools. Pace yourself, and take the first step.

You now have new information. Things will get better. It takes time and practice. Enjoy the process. All my best to you, as you find your way out of negative thinking and begin your climb up the ladder to Yes!

Vivian

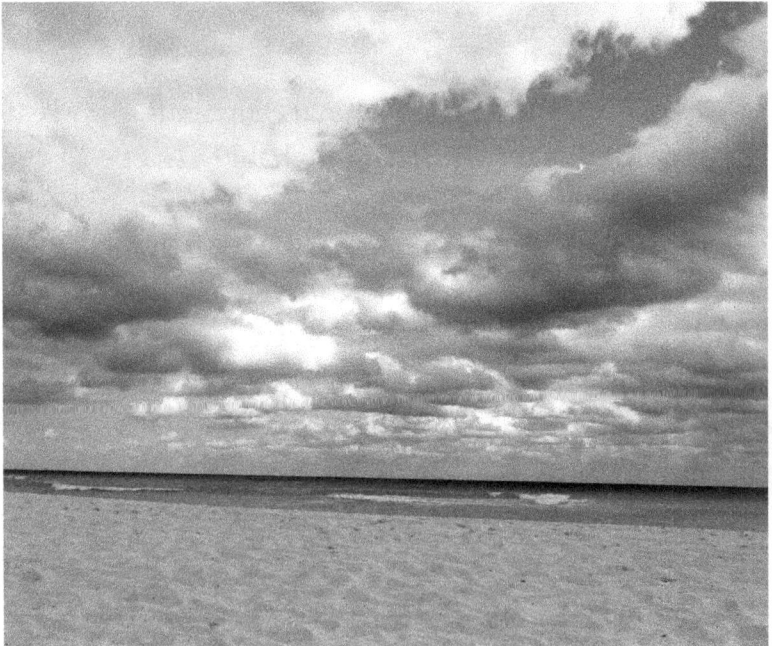

Vivian Orgel

PART VII

EXERCISES PROMOTING POSITIVITY

JOURNALING TO CLEAR YOUR MIND

There are no guidelines here, except to just write down what comes to mind, to help *clear* your mind, by putting thoughts down on paper. Instead of focusing on any negatives that appear, remind yourself that, by writing them down, you are releasing them.

_____

_____

_____

_____

_____

_____

_____

_____

_____

_____

_____

_____

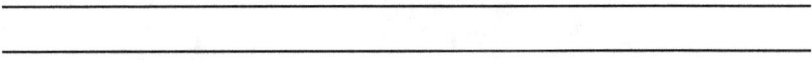

WRITE THREE OR MORE POSITIVE WORDS, FOR EVERY LETTER

Remember how the new studies show we may need to focus on three or more positive words in order to cancel out the effects of every negative word we see or hear?

For the next month, try to fill each letter page that follows, with positive words that begin with that letter. You might want to tack or tape the pages somewhere you are likely to see them often during the day. Each letter begins with a flower that starts with that letter and a few other words (and their definitions) you may not have heard of or hear spoken often. See how many other positive words you can think of, to add to each list.

You may want to look back through the book to find positive words in bold within the text.

(You can fudge on "X" if you like, using words containing the letter or sound of "X," for example: excited, exuberant, ecstatic.)

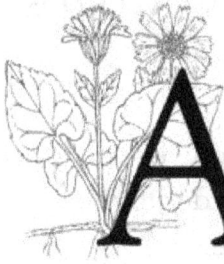

A ARNICA (Heart -Leaved) - A healing herb with bright yellow flowers.

Also:

ABSOLUTELY; ACCOLADE—award; ADEPT— thoroughly proficient; ARCADIA—scene of simple pleasure; AUBADE— song or poem, greeting the dawn; ABRACADABRA—magical charm

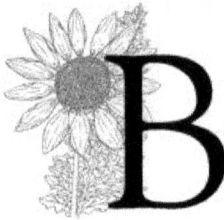

_____

_____

_____

_____

_____

B BALSAMROOT- In the sunflower family, it has bright yellow flowers & edible seeds

Also

BOUNTIFUL—plentiful; BOOGIE —get going or move to music; BENSON—blessing; BELVEDERE—beautiful view

_____

_____

_____

_____

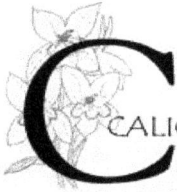

CALICO FLOWERS – Blooms are purple & white, and they attract butterflies.

Also:
CHARISMATIC; CRACKERJACK—marked by excellence; CARPE DIEM—seize the day; CHILL OUT—calm down. take a break; CHUTZPAH—extreme self-confidence; CUSHY—pleasant; CUP-of-TEA—something likable; CURATIVE—healing

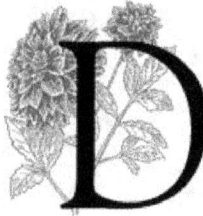

_____

_____

_____

_____

DAHLIA – It's easy to grow and creates a dazzling variety of colors - one called "crazy love."

Also: DELIGHTFUL; DAUNTLESS—fearless; DAZZLE—impress; DOWSABEL—sweetheart; DAYDREAM—wishful creation of imagination; DIVERSITY—variety; DANDY—fine

_____

_____

_____

_____

173

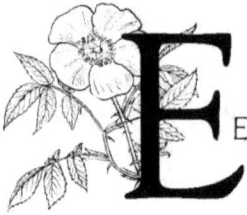

EGLATINE - An old world rose with white or deep rosy pink flowers.

Also:
EARTHSHAKING—momentous; EASYGOING—relaxed;
ELYSIAN—
blissful, delightful; EDULCORATE—make acceptable, soften;
EFFLORESCE—to bloom; EDIFY enlighten

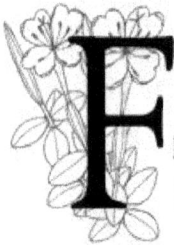

_____

_____

_____

_____

FIREWEED - has rosy or purple flowers that attract honey bees and humming birds.

Also:
FANTASTIC—great; FELICITATE—make happy; FACETIAE—
witty saying; FROLICSOME—playful; FARANDOLE—a lively
dance

_____

_____

_____

_____

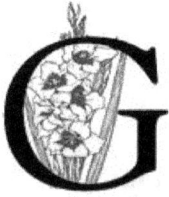

GLADIOLA – Sometimes called the sword lily, it comes in a wide range of colors, pastel & primary, and is called "glad" for short.

Also:

GRATITUDE; GUMPTION—enterprise, initiative; GRIT— courage, strength of character; GALORE—plentiful; GET-UP-AND-GO— energy; GALLIVANT—travel for pleasure; GEMUTLICH—pleasant and cheerful

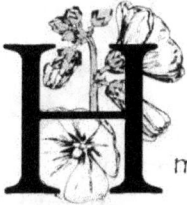

_____

_____

_____

_____

HOLLYHOCK – grows tall, blooms in many colors & attracts bees and butterflies.

Also;

HAPPY; HUMDINGER—extraordinary person or thing; HIP— Aware; HEAVEN-SENT—providential; HORIZON—attainable; HARMONIC—pleasing to the ear; HEY PRESTO—as if by magic

_____

_____

_____

_____

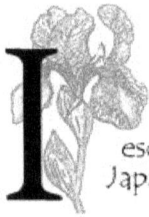

I IRIS –Named after the Greek Goddess who escorted the desceased to heaven & revered in Japan for its ability to purify negative engergies.

Also:

INGENIOUS; INCULPABLE—blameless; IDEATE—form an idea; ILLUMINATE—enlighten; IMPASSIONED—showing great warmth; INDUSTRIOUS—zealous; IDYLLIC—picturesque

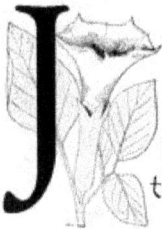

_____

_____

_____

_____

J JIMSON - One of Georgia O'Keeffe's favorite flowers to paint, also known as the moon flower because it blooms at night.

Also:

JUBILANT; JUICY—interesting; JITTERBUG—a lively dance; JACK-OF-ALL-TRADES—a versatile person; JAKE—fine

_____

_____

_____

_____

_____

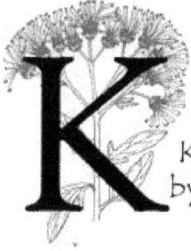

K KNAPWEED – An edible wildflower, loved by birds, bees and butterflies.

Also;

KINDNESS; KEEN—wonderful, alert, brave; KEMPT—trim, neat; KALEIDOSCOPE—display of changing patterns and colors

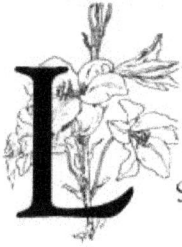

_____

_____

_____

_____

L LILY – Depending on its color, this flower is a symbol of purity, beauty, passion & gaeity & important in art and literature.

Also:

LOVELY; LAID-BACK—relaxed; LARGE-HEARTED— generous, sympathetic; LAUREATE—honor recipient; LIGHT-HEARTED—free from care, worry; LITHE— graceful

_____

_____

_____

_____

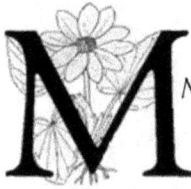

MARSH MARIGOLD- Unlike others, this marigold looks more like a buttercup one that floats carefree, like a waterlily.

Also:

MAGNIFICENT; MAFFICK—celebrate with rejoicing; MANNA —unexpected source of satisfaction; MAMBO—lively dance; MAVERICK—independent person; MAIN SQUEEZE—principal romantic person; MAGNANIMOUS—having a courageous spirit

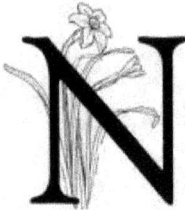

_____

_____

_____

_____

NARCISSUS - Named for its sedative quality, this flower is also a reminder not to take ourselves too seriously.

Also:

NUTRITIOUS; NIRVANA—bliss, heaven; NIFTY—very fine; NIMBLE—agile, sensitive; NEPENTHE something that makes one forget suffering; NO HOLDS BARRED— free of restriction

_____

_____

_____

_____

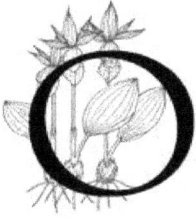

ORCHID (Calypso) – Often pink and magenta, this prized flower symbolizes joy, grace, royalty and admiration.

Also:

OUTGOING; OASIS—place of refuge; ODDS-ON—pretty sure; OLIVE BRANCH— goodwill offering; ORGUEIL—French for pride; OMNICOMPETENT—able to handle any situation; OPALESCENT—reflection of iridescent light.

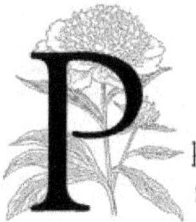

_____

_____

_____

PEONY - has many symbolic ties and healing qualities. It represents compassion, romance, prosperity, riches and honor.

Also:

POSITIVE; PACEMAKER—one who sets example; PERKY—self-assured; PALMARY—best; PLASTICITY—capacity to change; PALATIAL—magnificent; PERSEVERANCE—steadfastness; PLACID—calm

_____

_____

_____

179

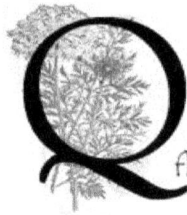

QUEEN ANNE'S LACE - A wild ancestor of the carrot, it is also called Bishop's Lace and Bird's Nest, because of the shape of its flowers. Its symbolic meaning is sanctuary.

Also:

QUALITY; QUANTUM—significant; QUALIFIABLE—capable; QUEENSHIP—regal quality; QUIESCENT=tranquil

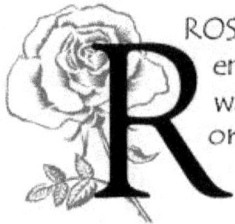

_____

_____

_____

_____

ROSE - Its colors run the gamut of positive emotions: red for deep feelings; yellow for warmth, caring; pink for joy, gratitude; orange for passion, energy; lavender for enchantment, love at first sight.

Also:

REBOOT—establish a new beginning; RACONTEUR—excellent storyteller; REGALIA—finery; REPLETE—very well provided; ROMANT—romance; RAZZMATAZZ—dazzle; ROMP—carefree play

_____

_____

_____

_____

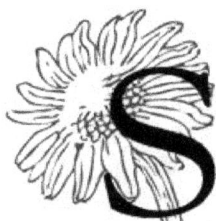

SUNFLOWER - It beams with warmth & positivity, its face always turned toward the sunlight, respresenting seeking truth.

Also:

SUMPTUOUS; SCINTILLATING—brilliant, lively; SIESTA—nap; SEDULOUS—diligent; SERENDIPITY—pleasant surprise; SPIFFY —fine looking; SHOW STOPPER—exceptional; SMOOCH—kiss

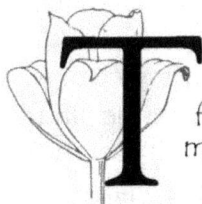

_____

_____

_____

TULIP - Valued for its simplicity, this flower represents perfect love and comes many varieties and colors.

Also:

TERRIFIC; TANTALIZING—stimulating; TEMERITY—nerve, daring; TERPSICHOREAN—having to do with dancing; TOUR de FORCE—feat of ingenuity, skill and strength

_____

_____

_____

_____

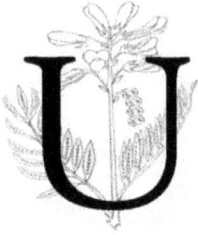

U UTAH SWEETVETCH – a wildflower, with pink, purple & white blooms, it's good for grazing & nourishes animals the air & the soil.

Also:

UNDERSTANDING; UNBEATABLE—not easily defeated; UNDER WAY—in progress; UP GRADE—improvement; UP-FRONT—forthright; UPROARIOUS—very funny

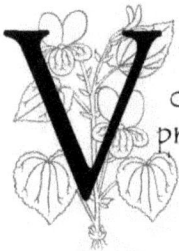

_____

_____

_____

V VIOLET – A flower with a long history of cultural & religious symbolism, it has healing properties & is used also as an edible decoration. It represents faith, true love & abundance.

Also:

VICTORIOUS; VALIANCE—strength of mind; VERVE— energy; VINDICATE—set free; VERACITY—truthfulness; VISIONARY— having foresight and imagination; VEHEMENT—passionate

_____

_____

_____

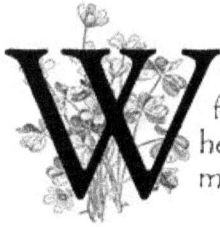

W WOOD SORREL – an edible plant, used for centuries by Native Americans for healing and nourishment. Its flower's secret meaning is joy.

Also:

WONDERFUL; WAMPUM—money; WASSAIL—go caroling; WHOOPEE—boisterous fun; WELL-BEING—state of happiness; WHIZ—wizard

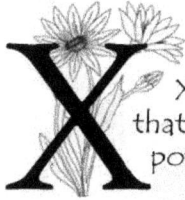

_____

_____

_____

_____

X XERANTHEMUM – A European flower that produces a fragrance believed to be a love potion and a dye that brings good luck.

Also

EXTRAORDINARY; XANADU—an idyllic or luxurious place; XYLITOL—natural sweetener that prevents tooth decay; XENIA—Greek for hospitality; EXPECTANT—looking forward to

_____

_____

_____

_____

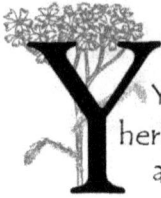

YARROW - Considered a sacred & medicinal herb, it is also a source of nutrition for birds & animals and brings diversity to landscapes.

Also;

YIPPEE; YES, YEA, YEAH, YEP—affirmative; YAULD—energetic; YOGA—exercise for well-being; YEOMANLY—loyal, brave; YEA-SAYER—person with a confident attitude; YOKEFELLOW—close companion; YLANG-YLANG—sweet-scented essential oil

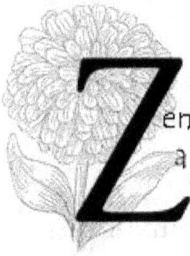

_____

_____

_____

_____

ZINNIA - A symbol of exuberance & endurance, this flower will bloom and brighten a garden for months. It symbolizes friendship and lasting affection.

Also:

ZEAL; ZAPPY—zippy; ZEPHYR—a gentle breeze; ZINGY—very appealing; ZAPATEADO—foot-tapping dance; ZUPPA INGLESE—sponge cake dessert; ZILLIONAIRE—very rich person

_____

_____

_____

Gratitude Journal

For the next 30 days, write down a few phrases each evening, reminding yourself of what you are grateful for.

Did someone show you kindness? Did you experience something of beauty? Did you have a delicious meal or enjoy something entertaining? How about that hug you got from your friend or the time you spent, playing with your pet? Did you get a moment to hear some sounds from nature or music you enjoy?

For example: "Today I sat outside, with the sun warming my face, and enjoyed the soothing sound of wind, rustling the in the trees. It was so relaxing and peaceful." Or, "A lot of what I needed from the grocery was on sale today!" Or, "I heard good news today; my friend is recovering from an illness." It doesn't have to be anything momentous. Most of us encounter numerous small gifts to be grateful for each day. When we focus on them with gratitude, they give us even more.

Day 1

_____

_____

_____

_____

_____

_____

_____

Day 2

_____

_____

_____

_____

_____

_____

Day 3

_____

_____

_____

_____

_____

_____

Day 4

_____

_____

_____

_____

_____

_____

Day 5

_____

_____

_____

_____

_____

_____

Day 6

_____

_____

_____

_____

Day 7

_____

_____

_____

_____

_____

Day 8

_____

_____

_____

Day 9

_____

_____

_____

_____

_____

Day 10

_____

_____

_____

_____

_____

Day 11

_____

_____

_____

_____

_____

Day 12

_____

_____

_____

Day 13

_____

_____

_____

_____

_____

Day 14

_____

_____

_____

_____

_____

Day 15

_____

_____

_____

_____

_____

Day 16

_____

_____

_____

_____

_____

Day 17

_____

_____

_____

_____

_____

_____

Day 18

_____

_____

_____

_____

_____

_____

Day 19

_____

_____

_____

_____

_____

_____

Day 20

_____

_____

_____

_____

_____

_____

Day 21

_____

_____

_____

_____

_____

Day 22

_____

_____

_____

_____

Day 23

_____

_____

_____

_____

_____

Day 24

_____

_____

_____

_____

_____

Day 25

_____

_____

_____

_____

_____

Day 26

_____

_____

_____

_____

_____

_____

Day 27

_____

_____

_____

_____

_____

_____

Day 28

_____

_____

_____

_____

_____

_____

Day 29

_____

_____

_____

_____

_____

_____

Day 30

_____

_____

_____

_____

_____

_____

Day 31

_____

_____

_____

_____

_____

~•~•~•~•~•~•~•~•~•~

    As another helpful exercise in gratitude, feel free to print copies of the following pages and fold them to use as a thank-you notes.

WITH SINCERE GRATITUDE

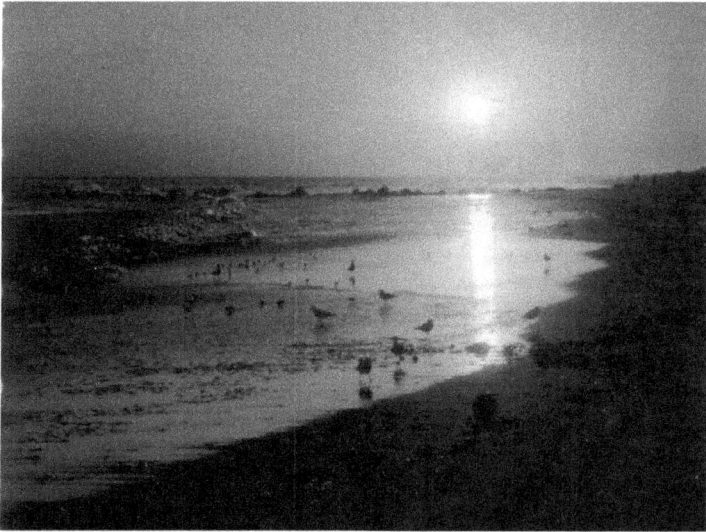

Vivian Orgel

THANKS SO MUCH!

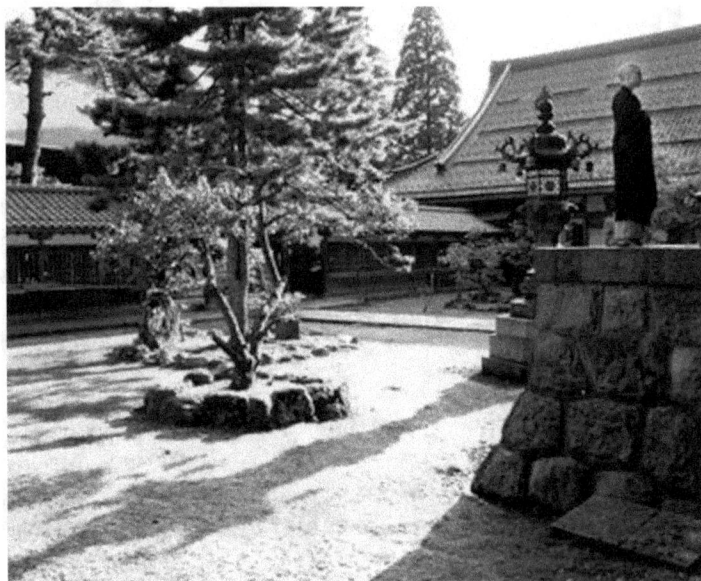

Micah Gampel

ACKNOWLEDGEMENTS

PAINTINGS

The paintings found at the beginning of each chapter were created by North Carolina artist, Henry Brown. Henry's life and art exemplify the power of positivity, in overcoming adversity and ill health.

Instead of giving up on life, after suffering a near fatal stroke a decade ago, Henry not only kept painting, but his style changed from realistic watercolor landscapes to the gorgeous and brilliantly colorful abstract style shown within, which Henry says his faith in God inspired. His ability in art was actually enhanced by what he and others are now seeing as his "stroke of genius."

PHOTOGRAPHS

Photographs in this book are contributed by Micah Gampel and Vivian Orgel. The book's cover is Gampel's work.

Micah Gampel is a Canadian photographer, who has been living in Kyoto Japan for more than two decades. His passion for photography was inspired by his father's collection of great photo books, particularly of Picasso, by photographers Doisneau and David Duncan. Trying to imitate them at the mere age of 12, using his first camera (a Kodak Brownie), he realized he had a natural love and a talent for photography.

EDITOR

I am lucky that Susan Wells Vaughan found my advertisement, requesting an editor. She could have a PhD, but she and I match on one thing: a PHD that means pursuing healthy decisions! She is a very special woman, with a huge database of experience and knowledge, which never ceases to amaze me. Synchronicity at its best, Susan adds so much to my projects, and I am very grateful that she found me.

Resources for More Information on Topics Covered

http://www.attn.com/stories/2587/what-negativethinkingdoes-your-brain

http://hellaheavenana.blogspot.com/2009/10/yes-yokoonosyes-painting-that.html

http://happierhuman.com/the-science-of-gratitude/
http://www.happify.com/hd/cultivate-an-attitude-ofgratitude/

http://my.happify.com/o/lp27/?srid=unknowN

https://www.psychologytoday.com/blog/words-canchangeyour-brain/201208/the-most-dangerousword-in-the-world

www.brainhealthconsulting.com

[Paraphrased article by Marie Rowland, PhD, included with her consent.]
http://my.happify.com/home/my-track/

https://www.ncbi.nlm.nih.gov/pmc/articles/PMC3132 556/

https://www.theroc.us/'

http://www.greenmedinfo.com/blog/probiotics-reducenegative-thinking
 http://www.walshinstitute.org/

http://www.foodforthebrain.org/

https://www.brainhq.com

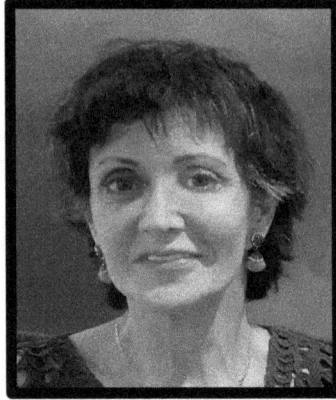

MindBodyBeauty.com highlights the philosophies of pioneering investigative author, Vivian **O**rgel, whose insightful opinions and research have been published in *The New York Times, Glamour, Self, Vogue, Essence, Seventeen* and many others. Her fact-packed, user-friendly website offers answers to the questions you have been looking for. It enlightens visitors by attacking myths from all angles, leaving only the exposed truth, regarding healthcare and cutting-edge surgical procedures.

Orgel focuses on issues that are constantly overlooked, to give the consumer an in-depth, astonishing glimpse into their skin care, hair loss and hair removal options. She is cited for connecting many underlying causes of and solutions to poor health, by bringing focus to advanced preventative measures for physical and emotional health.

She is a consumer advocate, as well as an educator for professionals in the fields of beauty and health sciences. Her philosophies and tension-management system offer healing from the inside and out. The **O**rgel Method is unlike any other, and it reflects Vivian's unconventional wisdom she shares to help others avoid needless trauma.

OTHER BOOKS BY VIVIAN ORGEL

To Help You Grow Wiser
and into the Best Version of Yourself

- Anger Management, Self-Punishment, and Second-Hand Stress
- Back Pain Management, Fighting Inflammation and Finding Quality Supplements
- Defending Yourself from Health Reducing Ailments
- 15 Methods to Hide Hyper-pigmentation and Dark Spots
- Holistic Methods to Change Skin Conditions, Discover Time- and Money-Saving Beauty Tips
- Home Remedies for Acne Problems: Getting Beneath the Surface
- How to Think Freely: Create the Downtime You Deserve
- Important Skin Care Information for Everyone and the Perfect Permanent Method for Hair Removal
- Negative Thoughts Don't Have to Own You: Enhance Your Career and Improve Your Health
- Physical Ailments…Ramifications and Remedies
- Preventing Emotional Eating: Eat Smarter
- Regaining and Maintaining Your Health
- Reprogram Your Mind: Save Your Skin
- Support, Motivation, and Inspiration
- What to Do About Your Skin's Stress Reactions to What You Tell Yourself: Experiencing and Eliminating Stress Perception

www.ingramcontent.com/pod-product-compliance
Lightning Source LLC
Chambersburg PA
CBHW060848280326
41934CB00007B/968